Praise for KSTechnique:
Healing the World One Person at a Time

"One of the most significant features of Kabbalah is how it integrates the physical and spiritual aspects of reality. In her groundbreaking work, Rabbi Jordania Goldberg has applied this unitive Kabbalistic principle to holistic healing. This book demonstrates how a modern healer can draw upon ancient mystical teachings and modern science, blending the two into an effective therapeutic system."
—DANIEL C. MATT, author of *The Essential Kabbalah, God and the Big Bang,* and the multi-volume annotated translation, *The Zohar: Pritzker Edition*

"Rabbi Jordania Goldberg has created a new healing modality utilizing energy healing, framed through the wisdom of Kabbalistic concepts. In this book she shares KST (Kabbalah Somatic Technique) with the world.

It is Rabbi Goldberg's mission to *heal the world one person at a time*, and in this book, she explains the way she uses kabbalah, physical technique and energy to yield a very powerful roadmap towards holistic healing—that of mind, body and spirit.

One can only be grateful for her insight, passion and dedication. May KST yield great success for Rabbi Jordania and the world!"
—RABBI STEVEN BLANE, Sim Shalom Jewish Universalist Synagogue

"Rabbi Jordania Goldberg has perfectly balanced profound principles of psychology with the oldest of spiritual teachings. In this book, Rabbi Jordania uses her deep, powerful, intuitive knowledge to apply Kabbalistic wisdom to holistic healing. This is a groundbreaking work that I would recommend to anyone interested in the healing arts."
—SUSANNA ADAMOVIC, MFT, Reiki Master, Private Practice in Santa Monica

KSTechnique
Healing the World One Person at a Time

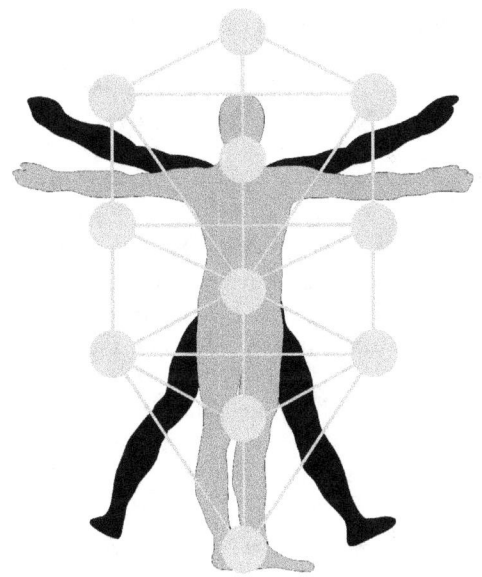

Rabbi Jordania Goldberg, MA, KSM

Las Vegas, NV

Copyright © 2020 by Jordania Goldberg

All rights reserved. No part if this book may be reproduced in any manner whatsoever without written permission except in the case of brief quotations embodied in critical articles and reviews.

Published and distributed in the United States by IPATH Inc., Las Vegas, NV.

For information contact:
www.kstechnique.com
www.ipath-inc.com
www.ipathcounseling.com

KSTechnique® is a registered trademark of IPATH Inc.

A portion of this book originally appeared in a different form online (2016).

ISBN: 978-1-7334153-0-9 paperback
ISBN: 978-1-7334153-1-6 ebook

Library of Congress Control Number: 2019911673

Editors: Gina De Roma, Dotti Albertine
Jacket and interior design: Dotti Albertine
Images: Rabbi Jordania Goldberg, Shutterstock, iStock
Author photo: Nikos Poulakis

Printed in the United States of America

First Edition

Part of the proceeds from the sale of this book go to:
Etz Hayyim Synagogue in Crete, Greece.

*This book is dedicated
to all the healers of the world:
that's YOU!*

CONTENTS

Foreword by Dr. Anne Weisman   *xiii*
Preface   *xvii*
Acknowledgments   *xix*

Part I / SEPHIROT

Chapter 1: **What is KSTechnique®?**   3
    Energy Constructs   6
    Role of the Observer   8
    Certification   11
    Ohrim   12

Chapter 2: **Breakthrough**   15
    ToL   18
    Reflection of the Multi-Verse   21
    Five Elements   24
    Five Phases of Materialization   25
    Kabbalah History   27

Chapter 3: **Sephirot** — 31
- Evolution of the Sephirot — 33
- Concept of Three — 36
- Sephirot as Energy in the Body — 38
- RT: Ruah Technique — 40

Chapter 4: **Malchut** — 45
- Grounding — 51
- Shechinah — 53
- King David — 53
- Quality of Earth as Matter — 54

Chapter 5: **Lower Triad** — 58
- Yesod — 60
- Hod — 64
- Netzach — 70

Chapter 6: **Upper Triad** — 77
- Tipheret — 79
- Gevurah — 85
- Chesed — 94

Chapter 7: **Supernal Triad** — 101
- Binah — 103
- Chochmah — 109
- Keter — 116

Chapter 8: **Sephirot Revisited** — 124
- Sephirot in the Body — 125
- Sephirot Body Map — 127
- The Pendulum — 131
  - How the Pendulum Works — 132
  - The Pendulum and the Heart — 133
  - Language of the Pendulum — 134
- Scanning — 136

Part II / HEALING TOOLS

Chapter 9: **Kavana** — 140
- Holding Space — 141
  - What is the Space we are Holding? — 143
- Unconditional Love — 144
- Energy Holds and Treatment Options — 144
  - Astrology and the Energy Hold — 146
  - Which Energy Holds and Elements? — 149
  - How Does Energy Feel? — 149
- What Makes a Healer? — 150
  - Professional Boundaries — 151

Chapter 10: **Protocols** — 153
- Procedure — 154
  - Remembering RT — 155
- Introduction to Sephirotic Script — 157
  - Script for Reading of Sephirot — 158
- Treatment Protocols — 161
  - Massage Table Protocol — 161
  - Seated Protocol — 162
  - Standing Protocol — 163
  - Spa Protocol — 165
  - KSH Protocol — 166
  - Foot Protocol — 168

Chapter 11: **Esoteric Anatomy** — 171
- Body of Asiyah — 176
- Body of Yetzirah — 177
- Body of Beriah — 178
- Body of Atzilut — 180
- Body of Adam Kadmon — 181

Chapter 12: **Healing Symbols** — 182
- Tetragrammaton as a Tool for Healing — 183
- Attunements — 184
  - Symbol Connections — 186
  - Activating Letters as Symbols — 186
- Lower Hey — 187
- Vav — 189
- Upper Hey — 192
- Yud — 193

Chapter 13: **Three Constitutions, Three Mothers, Three Symbols** — 196
- Three Constitutions — 202
  - Fire Constitution — 202
  - Air Constitution — 203
  - Water Constitution — 204
  - Attributes of the Three Constitutions — 205
  - Written Constitutional Assessment — 207
- Pulse Testing — 210
  - Pulse of Individual Sephirah — 212

Part III / MYSTERY

Chapter 14: **Angels** — 217
- Olamot and Angels — 218
- Temporary Angels — 219
- Archangels — 220
  - Archangel Michael — 222
  - Archangel Gabriel — 223
  - Archangel Uriel — 224
  - Archangel Raphael — 226
- Anthropomorphism — 227
- True Nature of Angels — 228
- The Fifth Element and the Angel Metatron — 229
- Working with Angels in Everyday Life — 230
- Conclusion — 231

Chapter 15: **Color** — **232**
- Definition of Color — 233
- Qualities of Color as Pigment — 233
  - Primary Colors of Pigment and Light — 234
  - Language of Color — 237
  - Hue of Computer Printing: Interpreting between light and pigment — 238
- Psychology of Color — 241
  - Color Keys — 243
- Frequency — 244
  - Frequency of Our Central Sun — 246
  - Tipheret as the Central Sun of ZA — 248
- Chakra — 249
  - ZA, Chakras and the Rainbow — 251
  - Are the Sephirot and the Chakras the Same? — 253
  - Merkabah, ZA, Chakras and the Body — 258
- The Rainbow and You — 258

Chapter 16: **Soul Traveling** — **259**
- What Is Soul Traveling? — 259
- KSMT — 260
- The Invisible Sephirah of Da'at — 261
  - KSH Protocol for Soul Traveling — 263
- CMBr — 264
- Merkabah — 268
- CMBr and KSMT Meditation — 268
- In Closing — 269

Part IV / CONTRIBUTIONS

Chapter 17: **KST Contributors** — **273**
- Sol Freidman — 273
- Gordon Goldberg — 274
- John-Reid Theriac — 275

Anne Weisman	277
Gina De Roma	277
Chapter 18: Case Studies	**278**
Anne Weisman	279
Aaron Nishimura	281
Danielle Gilbert	283
Eli Moran	285
Jordania Goldberg	286
Glossary	*293*
Bibliography	*301*
About the Author	*308*

FOREWORD

LEARNING KABBALAH SOMATIC TECHNIQUE® (KST) was the most incredible journey. When Joanne Hardy and I first began to work with this modality, I had no idea just how much this technique would impact my work, life and understanding. During that time, I was working as a massage therapist in hospice and in private practice. We had just wrapped up the first part of the training when I returned to work. As I entered the hospice to begin my shift, I saw the name of one of my home care patients on the list for our inpatient unit.

I prepared myself to begin my rotation and thought about trying this modality with him. I felt strongly that this would help. I saw his family in the unit and asked if I could work with him to do the massage and KST I was learning. They informed me that he was no longer responsive but that I could work with him.

I knocked on his door and introduced myself again as I entered the room. After I washed my hands and prepared for his session, I thought through the sephirot and began to work with him. As I moved through the sephirot and came up to Binah, Chochmah, and Keter, his energy was noticeably different. At Keter, he began to laugh gently and I almost hit the floor.

I let him know I was with him and doing massage and energy work, and at that moment, his father flew around the corner as he heard his son's voice. We gathered bedside as the patient spoke briefly and told us he was "just having the best dream." I told him to return to it if he wished. He smiled and slowly drifted off. His dad and I remained with him for the next few minutes. I finished the session and the enormity of what just happened began to settle in.

I completed my day in the unit, and as I was preparing to leave to go see my patients in home care, the hospice patient's nurse came into my office to let me know that he had just died with a smile on his face. I went to speak with his family and say goodbye. As soon as I was outside, I called Jordania to ask her what in the world did she teach me?!!?

I told her exactly what happened, and she listened in her beautiful way. From that day on, this technique has been an integral part of my practice. I use it with my clients, teach it to my students and meditate with it to discover what is happening in my own body. Through the years of doing this technique, many other incredible things have occurred.

Another person I encountered early in my learning of this technique was a friend who had recently been diagnosed with cancer. I was still learning the words and my Hebrew was rough. He patiently let me work with him as I placed flashcards on his sephirot and stumbled over the names and meanings. He has two children who watched and listened each day that I came in to do this work. They became my helpers and would place the crystals on their dad while we worked together. His journey through this particular bout of cancer led him out of state and it was then that we discovered that we could do this technique remotely.

I set up my table as though he was coming in for a treatment, and we picked the time to begin. I went through the whole session just as if he was laying on my table and the pendulum was picking up his energy! I took notes and recorded each reading. When each session ended, I called him and told him what the readings were. He and I were astounded as the readings were spot on. There was one particularly strange reading, in which the pendulum moved in a way I had never seen. We found out later that this was exactly where his cancer was. We did this work continually until he came back home and began to heal here.

KST is the most important modality I have learned. The applications for KST are broad and are useful in a variety of ways. Personally, I have worked with this modality through bodywork, guided imagery, meditation, distance energy work and in relaxation techniques. The information you will learn as you begin to work with KST is incredible. First, you will be able to connect with information held within your own body in a whole new way. Second, you will be able to connect with clients or patients at an entirely different level. You will learn ways to observe their energy within each sephirot while they are also becoming aware. Lastly, you will then be able to synchronize all of this information into an incredibly personalized treatment that will work on the mental, emotional, spiritual and physical bodies.

I hope you enjoy each page of the book you are about to read. As you soak in all of this information, relax into the synergies of the ancient wisdoms that are represented on these pages. Notice the elements from Ayurveda, Kabbalah, crystals, essential oils, bodywork and energy work that are interwoven in KST. Feel how this information changes your own perceptions and then watch as it changes those of the people you practice this with.

KST brings the interconnectedness of our being back into focus. This technique can heal our world, one person at a time.

DR. ANNE WEISMAN, PhD, MA, KSM, LMT is currently the Director of Wellness and Integrative Medicine at the School of Medicine, University of Nevada, Las Vegas. She is also a KSM level practitioner. While working as a massage therapist, Anne's work took her from spa and celebrity clients to hospice and stage four cancer patients. Her work at UNLV is helping transform our western model of medicine into a more integrative approach. Working with our world's future doctors gives hope that a holistic view of the body can become a natural part of the study of medicine. Anne's integrative, holistic approach to medicine continues to be an inspiration to those who work with her.

PREFACE

IF YOU HAVE CHOSEN TO PURSUE THE HEALING ARTS as part of your journey I hope the information found in these pages inspires you to continue.

KSTechnique® (KST) is a system of healing that bridges all other modalities—a Rosetta Stone of healing if you will. This book attempts to describe some of the philosophies learned and methods practiced by KST practitioners.

I thought it would take a few months to complete this book. The concept of KST was so simple in my head. Its inspiration came to me in a limitless second (albeit after decades of study and experience). A few years later I had written three short manuals, which I used for my teachings. Putting inspiration to paper was more complicated than I imagined.

The KST manuals are skeletal works that require lecture to complete them. Participants and I practiced this technique on our clients in the bodywork and counseling setting. It was intensely moving to witness the work. Those of us who had a background in the healing arts found it took our practice to the next level. Those who had no conscious experience with healing energy prior to performing this work began to report direct phenomena that was beyond what they were used to. Clients, likewise, reported benefits at an exponential rate. KST worked.

Teaching KST required small groups, in-person seminar settings, and the ability to check in with me directly. This meant limiting the number of individuals who could learn this technique. It was ideal. I could accrue valuable information about the efficacy of the technique while getting to stay in my treatment room and continue to be a comfortable, healing hermit.

Eventually I began writing this book as a way to answer the questions I was being asked about the work. It was taking years to write, but there was no hurry. My hope had been to publish this book and teach later after I retired. Then life happened, as it does. I was injured in a surreal pattern of events. Because of this I learned about the darker side of our social bureaucracy. I thought I was empathetic, but being crushed in this particular manner forced me to develop a deeper level of empathy for people no matter their circumstance. I've done my best to make that experience an exercise in maintaining a loving and neutral stance in life without being attached to the outcome: just like a healing session.

Following this last lesson, the first of two KST books is complete a bit earlier than I planned. What is that saying about the universe laughing while we're busy making plans? Let's allow the cosmic laughter to bring joy to our lives by letting it laugh with us as we traverse our roads of happy destiny.

May you receive infinite blessings and healings on your journey in life. Without a doubt, it is a journey worth taking.

—RABBI JORDANIA GOLDBERG, MA, KSM, Las Vegas, Nevada, May 31, 2019

ACKNOWLEDGMENTS

THERE ARE MANY WHO HELPED support the writing of this book.

I will forever be grateful to you!

My beloved husband Nikos Poulakis made sure I ate during my endless hours typing and retyping and made sure I never gave up. Dotti Albertine has supported me, no matter what, for over thirty-four years. She happens to be one of the best book designers in the country and was able to guide me in the writing and publication process of this book. Gina De Roma, is a dear friend of over thirty years, blogger, author of *Philosopher's Spoon*, yoga therapist, editor and KSM level practitioner. Her understanding of KST and her writing acumen enabled her to edit much of this book. My parents, Gordon Goldberg and e.l. Gordon were also wonderful during this time.

Jennifer Lynn, Joanne Hardy, Kala (Shannon) Stringert, Lynn Durkin, and Melissa Fielding, along with other KST practitioners, promoted my work in their spas where I was able to develop a deeper understanding of how KST works. Friends like Anja Zuckmantel, Anne Weisman, Bobette Vikan, Bryan Whittinghill, Cathy Tanner, Costa Derelis, Eilleen and Tom Raney, Dr. George Harouni, Jennifer Dixon, Jim, Sharon, Joseph, Catherine, John-Reed, Sileide, Jet and Leigh Theriac, Josephine, Sol and Jonah Friedman, Karen Simone,

Lance Takeo Izumi; Lori Cloutier, Mary Fossier, Mary and Eric Wright, Mickey Kaplan, Miguel Rivera, Perry Salit, Rabbi William Love, Rabbi Josh Katzan, Rabbi Malcolm Cohen, Snezana Adamovic, Tammy Scher, Trevor Dobbs, and Uriyah Zangen provided a wonderful, loving community where I could explore the ideas behind KST. I also wish to acknowledge the memories of Judah White and Bob Mataloni. May your memories be blessed.

There are others for whom I am so deeply grateful. You know who you are—especially on Monday nights!

Part I

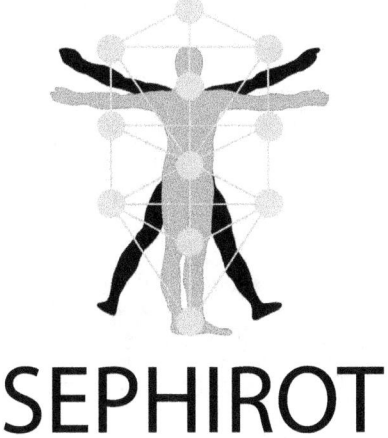

SEPHIROT

Chapter 1

What is KSTechnique®?

What lies behind us and what lies before us are tiny matters compared to what lies within us.[1]
—Ralph Waldo Emerson

KSTechnique® (KST) is a comprehensive healing modality. The letters "KST" stand for Kabbalah Somatic Technique. Based on the ancient practice of Kabbalah, KST teaches how each part of our body and mind has its own wisdom to share with us by offering a reflected portion of our greater innate wisdom—a microcosm of the macrocosm.

Rooted in the Tree of Life (ToL) and traditional Kabbalah, this profound technique bridges other modalities, including Ayurveda, Polarity, Reiki and Cranial Sacral, as well as scientific concepts such as Quantum Mechanics, Quantum Biology, Chaos Theory and Relativity. KST is a place where Kabbalah, other healing modalities, and modern science all meet. The words and approaches of each may differ on the surface. By decoding their respective terminologies and demonstrating the ultimate connection between these worlds, we find the similarities. KST becomes a key to understanding and utilizing multiple approaches to facilitating greater awareness for ourselves and others, a Rosetta Stone of healing, if you will.

A human being is part of the whole called by us 'Universe,' a part limited in time and space. He experiences himself, his thoughts and feelings, as something separate from the rest—a kind of optical delusion of consciousness. This delusion is a kind of prison for us, restricting us to our personal desires and affection of a few persons nearest to us. Our task must be to free ourselves from this prison by widening our circle of understanding and compassion to embrace all living creatures and the whole of nature in its beauty. No one is able to achieve this completely, but the striving for such achievement is in it itself a part of the liberation and a foundation for inner security. [2]

—Albert Einstein

Our research into modern forms of science is beginning to prompt us to rethink the orientation of the healing arts. The science of physics is defined as "the study of matter and energy and the interaction between them." The deeper our scientific understanding of these interactions the more we find a resemblance to the ancient healing arts.

KST can be described as a science of health rather than of disease, an approach that works with the whole person rather than the symptom. It can be deeply complex and rich in its teaching, or it can be as simple as learning to hold space with positive intention or *kavana*. Practitioners utilize KST as an energy medicine: a science that understands the body as an energetic aspect of the whole. Working with the healing power of the universal healing energy called *ohrim*, KST is the healing science that bridges past and future in the omnipresent now.

One of the reasons holistic healing differs from western technology, chemistry and other mechanical and medical research is that those involved with the latter fields of study often lost sight of the bigger picture of humanity as they explored the workings of our physical world and its inhabitants. In the past, scientists tended to see human beings and their surroundings merely as items to be viewed from the other end of a microscope. However, as those details have given way to a bigger picture within fields such as quantum mechanics, quantum biology, chaos and string theory (minus calculation issues), we are now poised to unite both the scientific and spiritual visions of the world into a more holistic vision of ourselves. We are not looking for a new science, rather we are looking to view ourselves and the universe through new eyes.

**We are already connected to the whole.
We merely need to shift our perspective to see it.**

The importance, as well as the shortcomings, of the specificity of science may be seen in a variety of circumstances. For instance, over the years, scientists in the fields of medicine and biology have categorized hundreds of diseases and a myriad of species. Although defining these categories helps us to communicate and express our individual observations and experiences, they are inadequate in representing the ultimate truth of a thing.

Likewise, the many tools and technologies for examination and diagnoses that have been invented during the last century have allowed for ever-increasing insight into the functioning of our bodies and the world around us. However, this clarification and insight into the various parts of our universe and ourselves has focused our attention on the individual trees of the forest, too often missing the intricacy of the whole.

The leaf is dependent on the life of the tree and the tree depends on the survival and health of the earth, air, and water that surrounds it. The leaf depends on the elements for things such as photosynthesis and fertilization. If we keep widening our circle of vision we see that the leaves and everything in the entire universe are interdependent. This exchange transforms fiery energy into warmth, water energy into moisture that gestates and creates, mental energy into the air that we breathe, and earth into the solid foods which provide nourishment to our tissues: all this emanating from the material of the cosmos.

KST emphasizes a shift in perspective that allows for observations of the world from wider and more varied angles. This means that the results, which from a narrower viewpoint may be seen either as psychic phenomena or miracles, need not be defined as such. When they do occur during the process of this work, results such as these are viewed within the context of a rational therapy that incorporates a wider interpretation of all systems of life, including the finer energy constructs. That allows us to touch realms beyond our physical senses.

ENERGY CONSTRUCTS

It is important to understand the workings of the physical body and mind when doing any sort of healing, bodywork or psychotherapy. Anatomy is what we study when we want to know about the structural composition of the physical body. Physiology is what we study when we want to know about how those structures interact within the body and mind. Psychotherapy is what we study when we want to know about the psychological composition of the brain and the mind-body connection. Once knowledge of these two primary systems is integrated, a greater awareness of the body and mind can be established.

The physical body itself can be seen as a collective which makes up an organism which we call human. This human organism, whether we are viewing it as "I" or as "other," represents a "whole." By dissecting its parts and systems we can better communicate, explore and understand the whole.

The energy field surrounding the physical body vibrates at a finer frequency than its physical counterpart, but both are still interconnected.

Einstein's famous formula, $E=mc^2$ (Energy equals mass times the speed of light squared) proved mathematically that mass and energy are related. Energy can be transformed into particles, and mass can be transformed into energy. A nuclear reactor demonstrates how matter can become energy, as do our bodies when we eat.

Since the physical body is composed of matter, and since matter translates to energy, then the study of physical anatomy, physiology, and psychology is a perfect foundation for the study of the energy field that extends from the body. Rather than considering them as separate, in KST the physical body can be seen as part of the esoteric anatomy. The other bodies of energy vibrate at a quicker frequency than our physical counterpart. The physical body is a denser form of energy.

Studying the structural anatomy and physiology of the energy fields is the same as studying it in the physical body, albeit less palpable most of the time. Separating the physical body from the energy bodies, or one energy body from the other, is simply a way for us to focus on a specific part, in order to better communicate, explore and understand the whole. In the same way that studying the anatomy of the foot helps us to understand its role in moving and supporting the body, focusing on a particular energy construct helps us to learn about and understand the whole that encompasses the human organism.

An energy construct is a section of anatomy, physiology or psychology of the energy field. The physical body is a part of this energy construct—esoteric anatomy, esoteric physiology and esoteric psychology.

Merriam-Webster defines the term construct in three ways:
1. to make or form by combining or arranging parts or elements—construct a bridge; construct a plan
2. to draw (a geometrical figure) with suitable instruments and under specific conditions
3. to set in logical order

In referring to energy constructs, we will utilize the latter definition. The term energy construct helps us to set in logical order particular parts of the esoteric or energy anatomy or physiology. When used as a general term we are directed to think about the structure of processes that govern the anatomy of a person when viewed as a field of energy. When used more specifically it directs us to study a specific section of that energy field.

For example, in KST, if we are working with an emotional block, we are directed to the Body of Yetzirah where emotional blocks are often held. If we then wish to talk about the energy construct that governs emotions generally, however, we can also see that emotional energy block connects to all of the other energy bodies. Narrowing our focus, we may see an extension of our original energy block corresponding to the limbic system (the physical area of the brain involved in emotional responses). This connection then relates to the emotional functions of the physical (Body of Asiyah), emotional (Body of Yetzirah), mental (Body of Beriah), through the causal (Body of Atzilut) and beyond. That emotional block, taken as a linear connection, or slice, among all of the energy bodies, would be considered an energy construct. This is why emotional blocks can be triggered by mental or physical phenomena when they relate or are connected to the emotional injury as part of the same energy construct.

That is also why an emotional block can affect all areas of our life, including our day-to-day functioning (Body of Asiyah). The aching of the emotions (Body of Yetzirah) generates mental fugue (Body of Beriah) and a disconnect from our sense of purpose in life (Body of Atzilut). Each body is part of a world that has a different frequency, association, framework and action. By utilizing the term *energy construct* we are able to set in logical order esoteric ideas, narrowing our focus of communication. This makes referencing their physical, anatomical and psychological counterparts simpler.

Each of these energetic constructs contains facets of consciousness, personality, relationship, stress, attraction and repulsion within fields of energy that may crystallize or slow in the body and become obstructions, distortions, judgments or disease.

The purpose of KST is to successfully integrate its practice with the knowledge of these systems in order to better prepare ourselves for working with others. It is like learning the map of a location we wish to visit. In this case, it is a map of ourselves in relationship to others and to the universe around us.

ROLE OF THE OBSERVER

CONTRARY TO WHAT IS OFTEN THE PERSPECTIVE of our emotional selves, we, as individuals, are not *the* center of the universe. We are each, however, viewing the world around us from *a* center of the universe. This center of our being, or soul, is one of infinite centers collectively belonging to the whole. Each of us views this whole from our unique location within the universe. As Einstein described in the quote that introduced this chapter, this singular perspective causes us to see ourselves as separate from the rest of creation. Our challenge is to widen our circle of understanding to embrace it in its entirety.

Using various KSTechniques, we can view flows of energy from the distinct viewpoint of our individual centers, and then widen that perspective to understand the relationship of those energy flows to the interplay of creation. By incorporating both the individual and the universal in our role as observers, KST gives us the tools to view health and illness as an interplay of energetic constructs. We begin to realize Einstein's vision of embracing all of nature in its beauty, as healer.

The KSTechnique® Practitioner

As practitioners of KST we understand the body as a field of energy. Utilizing the ohrim, which often emanates from the hands during sessions, the KST practitioner aims to balance energy fields, relieve tension and release blocks, bringing the body back into harmony with nature and the universe. By learning to hold space with clear kavana (intention), the practitioner can facilitate both energy balancing and healing.

KST provides a dynamic system of movement therapy, aromatherapy, chromotherapy, sound therapy, angel healing, cleansing, crystal work and health building, to name a few. Because this technique bridges many others, one could call it a Rosetta Stone of healing. It offers a profound body/mind/spirit psychology and a deep understanding of energy, nature, and the healing process.

KST offers a holistic, educational approach to healing. Practitioners furnish insight to those they assist, revealing a glimpse of the macrocosm reflected within the microcosm of the body. KST practitioners do not treat disease, rather, they support healing by providing resources which empower individuals to take responsibility for achieving their unique potential and accelerate their spiritual progression in a healthy, balanced way.

Whether within one session or across many, a Kabbalah Somatic Practitioner (KSP) shares techniques that promote awareness, health and balance. We each work with the client as a whole person, respecting the depth, integrity and choices they make on their journey toward evolution as a spiritual being. KST is a self-directed therapy that supports the client in recognizing and realizing their own higher level of inner guidance.

The Different Certification Levels of KSTechnique®

As a school, KSTechnique® has three certification levels. At the completion of each level, the practitioner will receive a designation of KSP, KSG or KSM.

Kabbalah Somatic Practitioner (KSP) is the first level and allows the practitioner to assess an overview of the systems of KST and to perform a cohesive treatment protocol.

The KSP level gives the practitioner the tools to perform and grow as a healer.

Level two is **Kabbalah Somatic Guide (KSG)** which reveals the worlds of energy at work behind the KSP tools. It is the difference between being a passive and active participant in the process of healing and growth. The curriculum for KSG level follows the same overall techniques found in the level one KSP program; however, the depth of material is far more extensive and detailed. Here the practitioner learns a deeper interpretation of the tools acquired in level one, as well as both the practical and esoteric reasons for utilizing those methods.

The practitioner begins the journey from student to teacher at level three, **Kabbalah Somatic Master (KSM)**. This level of study encourages a personal exploration within the system of KSTechnique®. Additional healing tools are provided as are the knowledge of the mechanics behind them, and the opportunity to develop a personal area of study. The contribution and process of this level allows the practitioner to contribute to the KST archives and to teach others.

CERTIFICATION

KSP consists of three separate twenty-five-hour seminars. Successful completion of these courses, along with fifty approved case studies, results in the practitioner receiving a KSP certification. The certification allows clients, employers and the healing arts community to understand that you have met the requirements set for this technique and have acquired the foundational and practical knowledge to perform it on clients.

During the first seminar, the practitioner will learn how to read the body's energy centers via the ToL and discover how this map impacts their life, as well as the lives of their clients. The practitioner can begin to see how the body, mind and emotions are linked and gains tools to work more in depth with them. The fundamentals of KST become tangible experiences rather than abstract concepts.

The second seminar focuses more on learning how the worlds of the esoteric anatomy make up the body. They are both a part as well as an extension of the physical body. The practitioner begins to see the body and the universe around it as vibrating to multiple frequencies of being, which are simultaneously autonomous and connected. By learning the esoteric anatomy of the *sephirot* and *olamot* bodies, practitioners begin to open new doors of exploration within the therapeutic setting and gain tools that help them work with these energies. This second seminar also provides additional tools to help balance this energy, including the use of sacred letters as symbols.

The third seminar explores how the body, emotions, mind and spirit interact with the ToL in a deeper way. We continue to explore those interconnections from the first and second seminars and learn how this knowledge can help us to connect with the environment around us. We begin to acquire more healing tools including distance healing, soul traveling and working with the energy of the angels.

KSG consists of a 500-hour program and 108 additional approved case studies. It is not necessary to progress to this level in order to provide KST to clients, as the information learned in level one is more than sufficient to perform a cohesive treatment and continue to grow as a healer.

The KSG level of study is intended for the practitioner who wishes a achieve a deeper knowledge of the mechanics of the KSTechniques gained in level one, as well as adding additional techniques to their toolbox.

It is often thought that the quality of mystery makes things more interesting. Ironically, the process of demystification which is provided in level two makes the ToL, ourselves and the universe around us that much more fascinating. The goal of the KSG level is to demystify the mystical which often requires more intense study and practice. That is what is accomplished here.

KSM trains the practitioner to communicate all of these teachings as a cohesive system that facilitates others in learning and beginning their own journey on the ToL. This level requires that the practitioner create an individual contribution to the KST archives by way of a formal project. Examples of KSM contributions include: Anne Weisman's distance reading technique and Gina De Roma's work on the relationship among *tarot* cards, *I Ching*, Kabbalah, KSTechnique® and yoga. Gina has also helped with editing the KST book and manuals.

By continuously incorporating the diverse insights and contributions of KSM candidates, the goal of KST is to remain an organic, co-creative tool for growth, *bittul* (egolessness) and enlightenment. As practitioners we seek to achieve our potentials in life and facilitate ever increasing opportunities for healing.

OHRIM

OHRIM IS THE UNIVERSAL HEALING LIGHT that is directly connected to the uppermost worlds beyond time, space and duality. The English language uses the Roman or Latin alphabet to compose words. Using this alphabet to spell the Hebrew word *ohrim* masks a deep mystery contained within the last letters of the word when spelled using the Hebrew alphabet. The *im* at the end of the word ohrim is a Latin alphabet shorthand for the Hebrew letters Yud and Mem. When spelled with the Hebrew alphabet, this suffix denotes both *the plurality that becomes one* and *the infinite connecting to the finite.*

Attunement with the unconditional energy of the ohrim is a lucid state which integrates the higher and lower frequencies of the body. It is a personal experience of exalted consciousness and enhanced well-being, which provides balance, clarity and personal integration. By facilitating this attunement, we hold the *kavana* (intention, direction of the heart) in which we can become a more conscious participant in our life.

The skilled practitioner utilizes these tools to provide for a more effortless expression of healing. We keep our *kavana* on the good of the whole. This universal perspective allows us to connect with the experience of *bittul*. Self-transcendence reminds us of the importance of keeping the ego in check so that we are freely able to become tools for healing and vehicles for the *ohrim* behind and within our universe.

As conduits of healing, we must always strive to keep ourselves in integrity as we push toward more learning and understanding. This dedication of *kavana* will aid us in fulfilling our potential as therapists, healers and conscious beings. By transcending the will of the self and surrendering to the universal intention, we allow the ohrim to move us past the limitations of our ego's experience and assist our clients in finding their own paths to health and personal fulfillment.

Chapter 2

Breakthrough

All beings are flowers blossoming
*In a blossoming universe.*³

—Soen Nakagawa

BASED IN THE ANCIENT STUDY AND PRACTICE OF KABBALAH, KST offers a comprehensive energetic approach to the healing arts. In this evolutionary paradigm, all forms of energy within creation and beyond are the expressions of an ever-evolving conscious universe. Life is understood as a learning experience for the soul. Our path between birth and death becomes a cycle of growth.

This sacred perspective suggests a deep respect for the individual and the depth of the human condition. Our growth and the challenges we face during the various stages of our life are a sacred journey. We embody every moment of an ever-evolving state that we call universe.

Every flower requires sunlight, water and nutrition in order to bloom, but the amounts needed of each of these requirements vary with the individual. Some flowers grow best in temperate climates and some bloom in what we might consider harsh surroundings. Everything we face in life, every challenge we face during our growth, anything we interpret as resistance to our actualization, can be seen as providing the optimum environment for our expansion. Each season we grow through is a movement in the unfolding of the evolutionary process.

KST dignifies the challenges we face in life and the diseases we encounter by understanding them in an evolutionary context. Disease is understood as an imbalance which occurs when the body's energy frequency decreases in a particular area in order to draw attention to it. These imbalances are sometimes an indication that the individual needs a space to rest, to regenerate, and to receive resources and support. Accidents and illness are sometimes an unconscious expression of issues that are too threatening for the ego to deal with consciously.

When we find it too painful to be present in our feelings, cells may contract and energy become blocked. A KST practitioner energetically holds space for the client to experience feelings. We create a space in which the client accepts that it is safe to be present in their body, safe to breathe, to be conscious and to be fully alive. The KST practitioner facilitates the clearing of trauma from the cellular memory of the body.

The above examples describe how the disease process develops due to personal imbalance. There are other cases that have nothing to do with the imbalance of the individual. These could be traced to ancestors, community or the world. During these times, we get sick because we are participating in the tikkun (rectification) process of the world. Imbalance is a part of the tikkun. When we are unbalanced we naturally seek balance. We draw stabilizing forces to ourselves. Likewise, in KST we would say that we uplift the frequency of the world through the transmutation of stuck energy.

Issues will come up when an individual is ready to meet them. The role of the KST practitioner is to assist in bringing these issues to conscious awareness so that the client has an opportunity to fully participate in the healing process.

During the first level of KST the practitioner learns to read the ToL in the body in order to assess what is out of balance. Once the imbalance is assessed, the KST practices of healing can ease the release of tension, resistance, and body armoring by helping to quicken decreased frequencies in the body.

Within this role, the KST practitioner holds an attitude of deep respect for the client. The practitioner is trained to know that creating space for healing means providing an environment where the client can participate at their own pace in a way that honors their divine and unique path in life.

Frequency is the measurable manifestation of the universal animating force. In chapter one, we defined *energy constructs*. We saw that Einstein's famous equation demonstrates how matter and energy are equivalent to each other. We discussed how the physical anatomy and its esoteric counterparts are parts of the energetic body as a whole, each vibrating at a different frequency. The understanding of frequency is drawn from a broad range of esoteric philosophies and science but grounded in KST. *(See illustration below.)*

The Senses

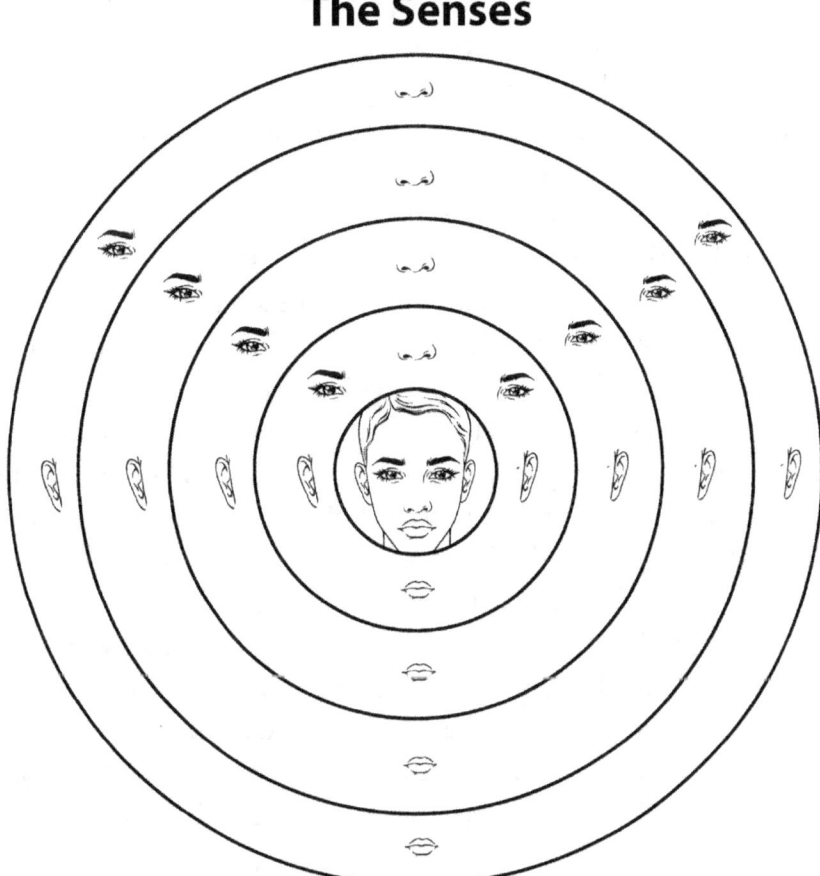

Chapter one introduced us to the universal healing light known as ohrim. It explained how attunement with its unconditional energy can integrate the higher and lower frequencies of the energetic body. Our attention is directed to the ToL within the body with the ohrim as our guide.

ToL

ToL MEANS THE TREE OF LIFE. Whether as a term or an image, the ToL can be found and explored in countless religions, spiritual paths, philosophies and sciences. It represents and describes the building blocks of the creative structure that is everything. It is a holographic world of wonder that allows us to experience our lives as separate even as we are simultaneously connected to all.

Each ToL is composed of ten sephirot, emanations of the infinite. They are expressed as spheres on the geometric representation of the ToL. These spheres are called sephirot. Their names are: Keter, Chochmah, Binah, Chesed, Gevurah, Tipheret, Netzach, Hod, Yesod and Malchut. Each will be explored in greater detail in other chapters. *(See illustration on the following page.)*

There is a ToL that spans our known universe, one for the universe above that and so on. Living matter is a reflection of the ToL. Every aspect of creation has its own ToL. They facilitate the functioning of our bodies as well as each cell within our bodies. *(See illustration on page 20.)*

At the nucleus of every atom, molecule and cell of the body is an energy field of a higher potential that is in tune with the spiritual realm. The physical field is a radiation from this spiritual nucleus. It is the body's attunement with the ToL that sustains its physical life. The ToL helps in the manifestation of the body as a vehicle for life.

This magnificent form of the ToL is the foundation of every structure, great and small, organic and inorganic. It offers us a framework of study. Through it, we explore the worlds around us and within us. This framework supports and grounds us in our exploration until such time when we reach a level of awareness where we are comfortable with living

ToL / Ten Sephirot

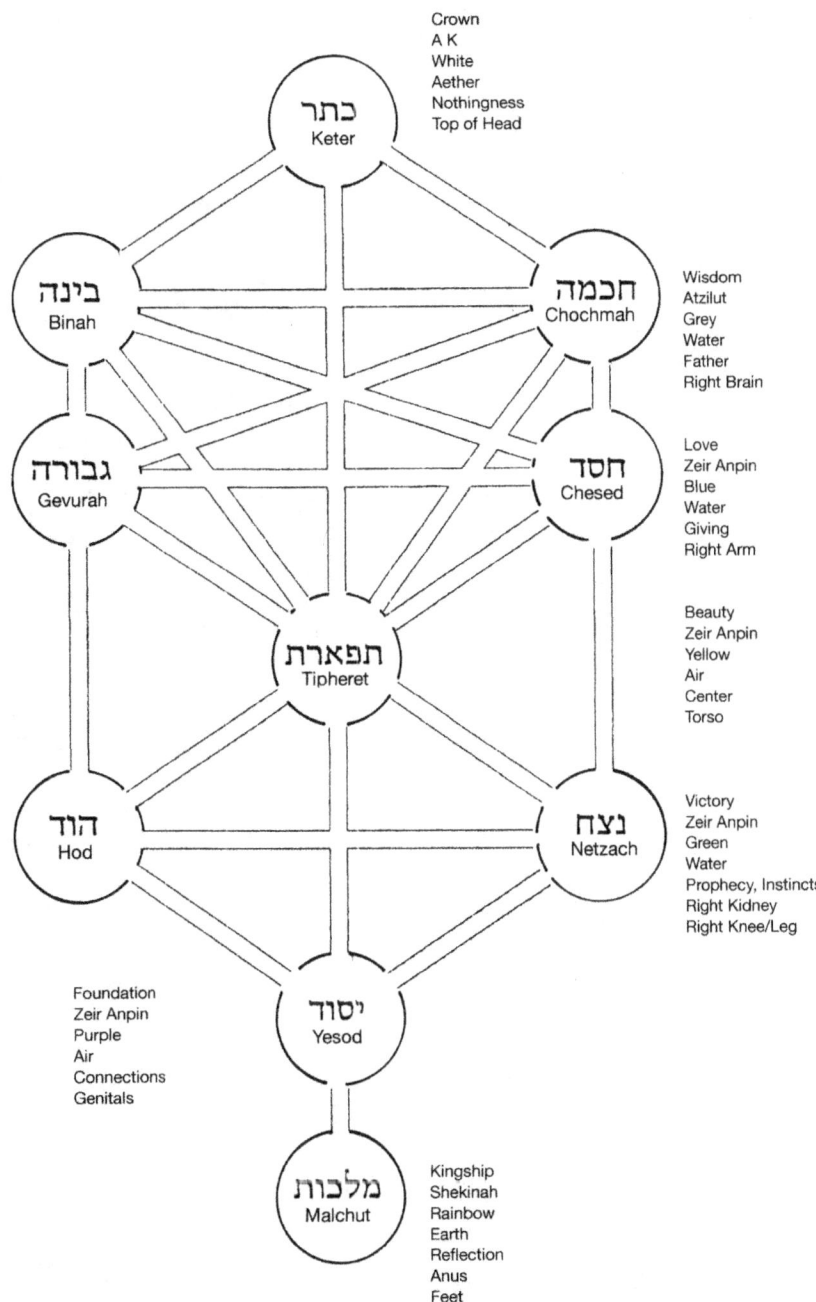

FIVE LEVELS OF THE OLAMOT WORLDS
Tree of Life for each world. Tree of Life for all life.

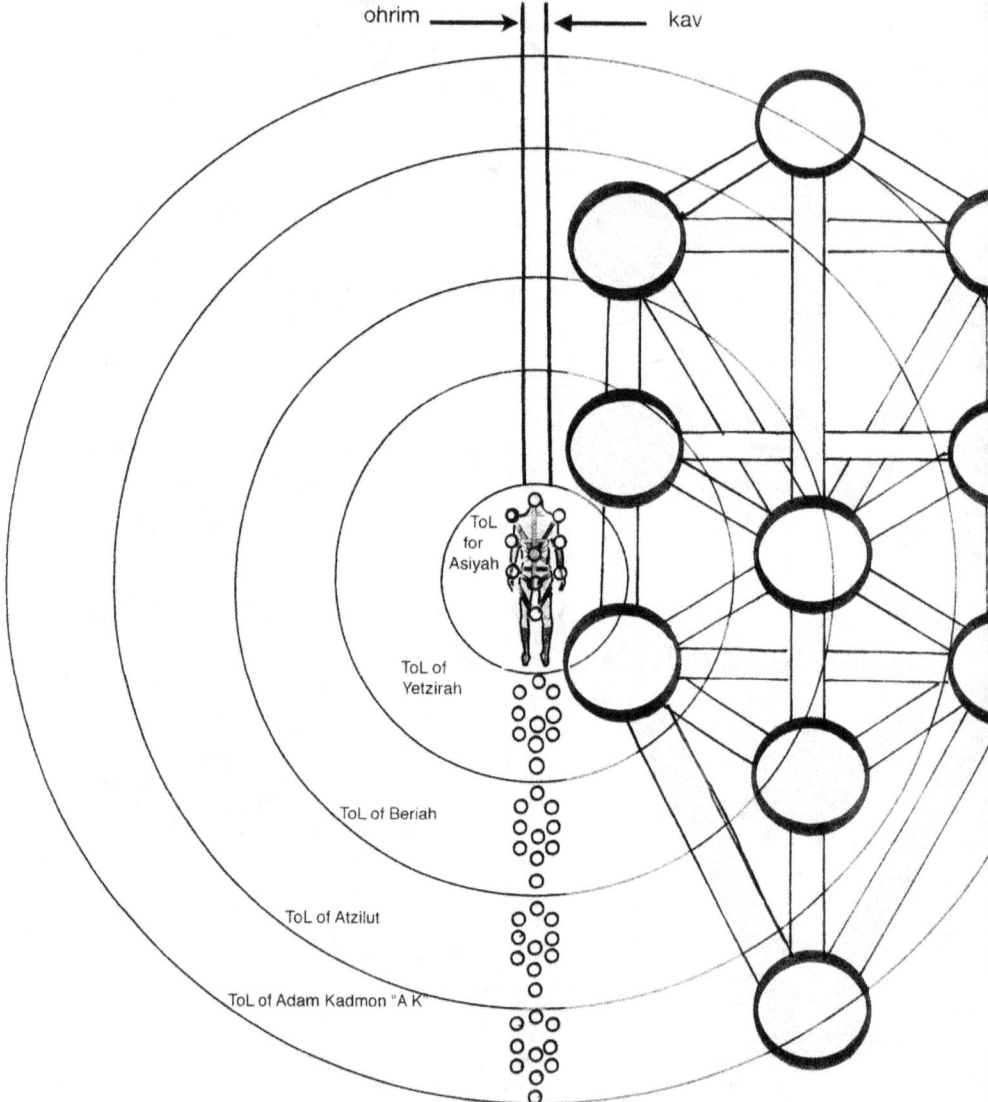

in our body and experiencing its infinite connections. We maintain the balance necessary to live life on life's terms.

Our goal is to find the sublime within the mundane. We connect with the divine even as our feet firmly walk the earth of our daily lives.

As Gurumayaji once advised, "It is much easier to meditate while sitting on a balanced checkbook."

REFLECTION OF THE MULTI-VERSE

WE EXIST IN A MULTI-DIMENSIONAL UNIVERSE.

Modern science speaks of dimensions, frequency and the breakdown of Newtonian thought processes. Kabbalah speaks of the dimensions of the sephirot and olamot worlds. These support our understanding of the healing process. We incorporate the energetic frequency of the ohrim and a non-Newtonian explanation for how our universe was initiated. Kabbalah and cosmology both describe the process of creation in different ways that, for the purposes of KST, have the same meaning.

As will be detailed further in chapter eleven, "Esoteric Anatomy," our energy bodies are mirrored within the five olamot worlds and the ten sephirot that compose creation. These form a blueprint for our esoteric anatomy.

As we learned in chapter one, the ohrim is a universal healing light which is directly connected to the uppermost worlds. By exploring the *Map of Avir on page 25* we can follow the path of the ohrim from its source along the path of creation. This is a path that is simultaneously an origin story and a description of an ongoing, living expression.

From the physical perspective of Asiyah, the universe can be understood, not as a static, fixed place in time and space, but rather as an evolutionary process: the unfolding of creative potency. We will describe this path in historic terms, but this process is a continuous one.

Although we utilize scientific language here, our description of the ohrim's creative journey is given from a metaphorical perspective, as modern science—at the level of Asiyah. We currently lack the concepts and terminology to completely describe creation that emanated from realms which vibrate higher or lower than our human brains and modern devices are capable of deciphering. That said, since we will use a couple of scientific terms in our description of the ohrim's path, a brief definition of those terms may be helpful.

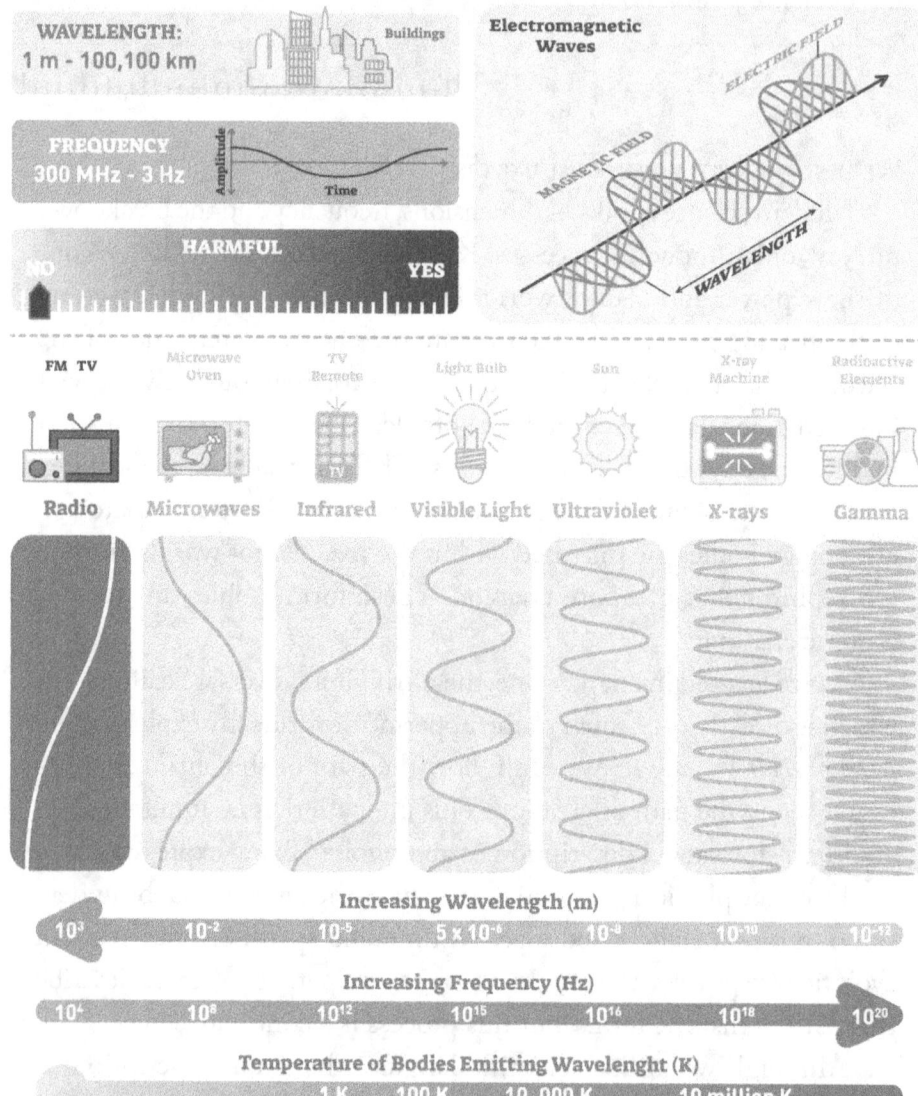

Frequency is a property of waves. A wave is a vibration that carries energy along with it. Just as an ocean wave carries a surfer along with it to the shore, if you are hearing this chapter read aloud, the voice of the speaker is coming to you as sound waves. Frequency is measured as the number of times a point on a wave passes a fixed reference point in one second. An exception would be the human heart beat, which is measured in beats per minute. As frequency increases, wavelength decreases and vice versa. Again, if you can picture ocean waves heading towards the beach, higher frequencies have shorter wavelengths and lower frequencies have longer wavelengths. The water moves at the same speed, but the shorter waves pass by a particular grain of sand on the beach with greater frequency.

Light is an electromagnetic wave. There are electromagnetic wavelengths that we are unable to see with our human eyes. They include: radio waves, microwaves, infrared, ultraviolet, x-rays and gamma rays. Certain sound wave frequencies that the human ear cannot hear also exist. KST describes worlds which vibrate at wavelengths above our physical awareness, such as the those from which the ohrim originated.

Attenuation is a term that describes a gradual loss of intensity or quantity as something passes through a medium. For example, ear plugs attenuate sound coming into your ears; lead attenuates x-rays and water attenuates both light and sound. When the light of the sun reaches the sea surface, the intensity of light decreases exponentially with the depth of the water.

The healing, guiding frequency of the ohrim originally radiated from the highest spiritual realms of Atzilut, Adam Kadmon, and beyond. From its origins as pure light (Ein Sof)—manifesting as the kav (pure light in action), via numerous contractions of the light—our universe, with its olamot worlds, was birthed. As the light progressed downward from these upper worlds, its frequency was attenuated, creating lower worlds, each vibrating at a seemingly reduced frequency; creating and transforming as those planes of existence came into being. They culminated in the lowest frequency of our physical and material realm of Asiyah.

This energy on every level of creation continuously moves through this evolutionary cycle and is conscious on each level as an extension of itself. Our soul exists on all these levels at all times. The ohrim then expresses through the fundamental forces of nature (the five elements). These elements have a vibratory basis which underlies the universe. They coordinate within our body/emotions/mind as elemental constitutions.

The evolutionary course of this path helps the ohrim express the essence of intelligence. It is a cycle of universal healing light moving from a source out into creation. We experience the ohrim as a field flowing through us and returning to the source.

All energy moves in this circulation of intelligence. The journey is a movement from a neutral source to a positive field, then through a negative phase, returning to neutral. This cyclic pathway follows the triads represented in the ToL which is mirrored in most other disciplines. It is the caduceus of western medicine, the doshas of Ayurveda, the Three Mothers of Kabbalah and the constitutions of KST. They form the basis of treatment in KST and create a path for us to follow on our way to fulfilling our potentials in life.

FIVE ELEMENTS

FROM THE DAWN OF OUR WRITTEN HISTORY the five elements were understood as archetypal forces that continue to be mirrored in the modern science of today. They are: aether (space), air (gas), fire (heat), water (liquid) and earth (solid). Their elemental energies radiate throughout, as our bodies and universe, connecting us with everything that is, was and will be. They descend from the highest of frequencies and permeate every cell and conscious intent of existence, stepping down from spirit as solid matter through five phases of materialization. Each of the elements is a world unto itself. All energy in our physical world of Asiyah is attuned with these five elements and each is reflected in the five layers, or worlds, of creation *(See following Map of Avir.)*

In its journey from the highest realms to the material, the potency of the ohrim seemingly drops as the energy goes from aether to earth. But this is indeed a play of illusion in creation. For as the frequency is attenuated and decreases, the potency becomes coalesced as matter. To touch the core of matter is to touch the power of the original frequency of creation. All creation, as vibration, is sustained by its reflection as these elemental forces within Malchut. In this way, the five elements sustain the five phases of materialization.

Map of Avir

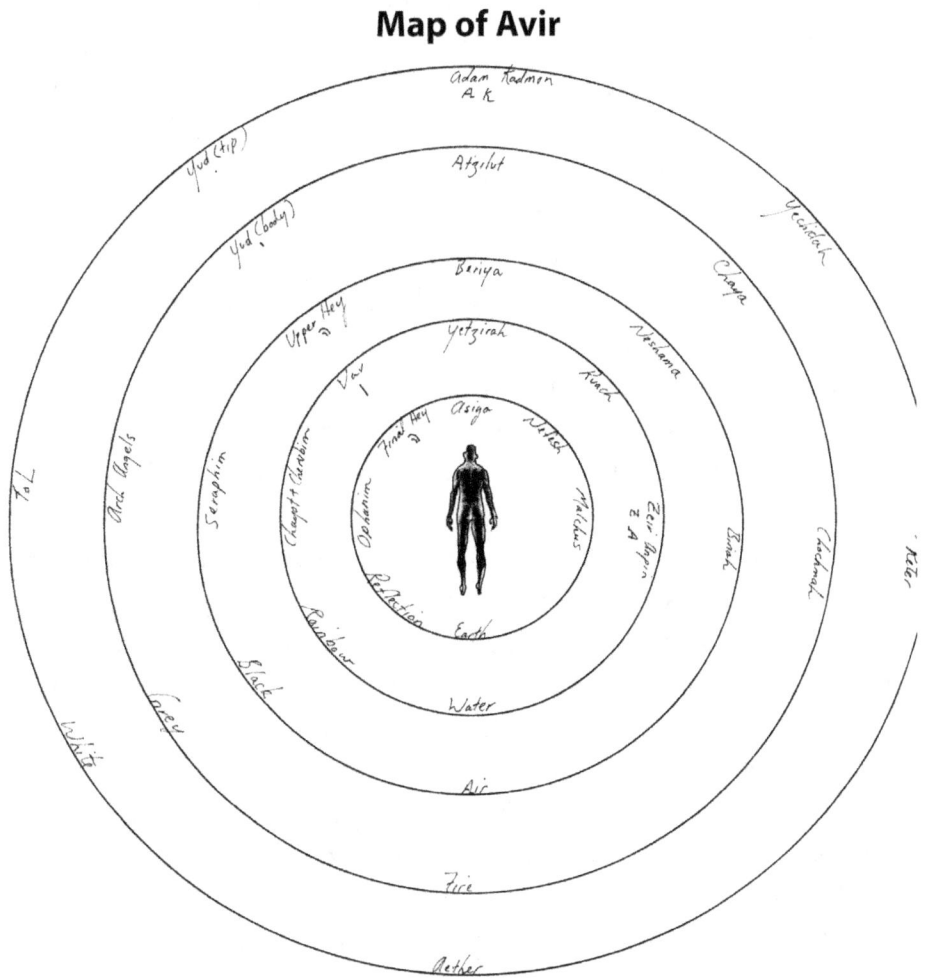

FIVE PHASES OF MATERIALIZATION

ALL ENERGY BEGAN FROM THE HIGHEST OF FREQUENCIES as the light of Adam Kadmon. Then the frequency lowered, becoming fire, as the electromagnetic force, and establishing the World of Atzilut, where the potential for time and space can be found—where past, present and future exist as one. The frequency attenuated further via the kav, becoming air or wind, as the weak nuclear force, and Beriah was established. Then it continued to lower and decrease, expressing as the water of Yetzirah and the strong nuclear force. It then flowed life into Asiyah, where it expressed as earth and gravity. These five elements create the structure from which the creative expression and universal life force of the ohrim can express itself.

Our physical sense organs are tuned to the dimension of matter, or level of Asiyah, where vitality is the source of our aliveness. On this level, our vitality is what we sense. Within that vitality is our spirit or ruah, which envelops our soul or Nefesh. Such is the anatomy of Asiyah and our physical awareness. It comprises but a small percentage of the whole of the reality that is us: those parts that are outside the cycle of birth, death, and decay. When our spirit leaves the body, so does our soul. The corpse that remains begins to decompose immediately as it goes back to the world of physicality.

The impressions and experiences of the physical and the Body of Asiyah do not disappear into the oneness. Rather they are infinitely imprinted on the soul itself. The physical body and its corresponding bodies found on higher levels do not disappear upon decommission. Their imprint on the soul is continuous and infinite. It is the ongoing interplay between the highest levels, where all things have occurred, will occur and are occurring on our human level of existence. Here, free will results in a rich transformation of soul and experience.

Just as the sensory organs of reception of the nose, ears, eyes, mouth and skin exist and experience Asiyah, so the nose, ears, eyes, mouth and skin extend their frequency to match that of the next level of Yetzirah in order to perceive on that level. All these sense organs are connected. So when we shift our consciousness to the higher frequency of Yetzirah we are sensing through expressions of our physical sense organs that already exist there. Our various energy bodies, known as the avir, are thus a part of an all-pervasive field of awareness that extends throughout infinity.

We do not need to die in order to access the other levels of our avir or energy bodies. We need but shift our consciousness to the frequency of another dimension or world in order to access the information being gathered there by our organ senses that exist on that plane. This is what is commonly referred to as extrasensory perception. This often-mysterious source of information can readily be understood as a basic part of the esoteric anatomy of the avir.

Oneness is the foundation of this cosmology. In this ancient wisdom reborn, there is an understanding of the identity of all consciousness. Each of us possesses an individual awareness that is but a drop within an ocean of consciousness which, itself, is one with oceans beyond.

Similarly, every element of creation contains its own ToL. Each ToL is one with all life, all awareness and beyond. The ancient wisdom is rooted in the understanding of the oneness of all consciousness and the sacredness and unity of all life. The changing world of appearances is an emanation from an unchanging universal field of living intelligence. As practitioners we hold space for this infinite intelligence and invite the universal healing energy of the ohrim to heal and connect us to our greater whole in health and healing.

Our earth, nature, solar system and our bodies are part of a single system of creative intelligence. All life systems are subsystems of the evolution of the one life of the universe. Ohrim, the universal healing light, is present in every part of our body, emotions, mind and spirit. The material body is an emanation of this energy. Our attunement with the ohrim is the key to unlock the healing and health that can be found across worlds of consciousness and light.

KABBALAH HISTORY

KABBALAH, A POETIC SYNTHESIS of spirituality, science and metaphysics, is the foundation for healing in KST. It offers a "Rosetta Stone" of healing. Its basis is the oldest of the healing traditions. This mystical teaching has been a source of knowledge for thousands of years. In that spirit, it is important to explore a bit about the history of traditional Kabbalah here.

As Kabbalah evolved and its spirit moved through the centuries its wisdom was only taught as an oral tradition. It was passed from one initiate to the next, using the strictest of guidelines and adhering to complete secrecy.

The oral tradition found its way into written literature during the last couple of thousand years. Some examples are the 13th century, Kabbalists, such as Moses de Leon, who published the Zohar (Inner Light) after ascribing it to Shimon bar Yochai (Rashbi), and Chaim Vital, who transcribed the teachings of the Ari (Issac Luria) in the 16th century as well as the Bal Shem Tov in the 18th century. This period marks an enriching movement in Kabbalist history.

During the second temple and Bar Kochbah times, writing down a previously protected oral tradition had become necessary in the face of the persecution and killings of Kabbalists. To not write these teachings down would have meant the potential annihilation of many great and ancient works.

Kabbalah includes a mythology that is traced back to the patriarch Abraham, who is credited with having composed great Kabbalistic works, including the oral version of the *Sefer Yetzirah*. Abraham's sons, born of his second wife Hagar (Keturah), were sent to the East with many gifts, bringing with them the knowledge of Kabbalah. Their arrival in the East may have influenced the philosophy of the Vedas in India where Ayurveda, which contains information on the chakras and yoga, is found. Since the trade routes between Mesopotamia and the East, including India, were well traveled during the time of Abraham, it is likely that this is the case. Thus, whether it be Abraham as a singular entity, or a collective community, this wisdom could easily have traveled between the West to the East.

Likewise, such books as *Sefer Razial* are attributed to the oral tradition of Adam, hinting that this education began with the dawn of humankind and is an inherent part of us. In that way, Kabbalah becomes the study of our own being and our place within creation. Historically these literary works can be traced to writers who lived well after Abraham was said to have lived.

The influence of Kabbalah on other philosophies, medicines, healing modalities and sciences is evident. For example, the similarities between the Vedic and Kabbalistic systems are apparent on many levels. A Vedic concept like reincarnation may be likened to the Hebrew teaching of Gilgul HaNefesh, the cyclical reincarnation of the wandering of the soul. Karma, the "imprinting" carried from a previous lifetime, reminds one of the Hebrew hashgacha pratit, the specific cause-and-effect relationship molded by past lives. The tests and openings that constitute moments of opportunity to change the destiny of one's reincarnation are called bardos in the East and nissyonot in Hebrew. Hindu prana and the Qi of traditional Chinese culture are comparable to the concept of Ruah HaKodesh. In keeping with this kinship, KST level II explores the various levels of creation and the human energy fields found in Kabbalistic teaching that are beautifully reflected in the auric system of Ayurveda.

The most beautiful thing we can experience is the mysterious.
It is the source of all true art and science.[4]
—Albert Einstein

In our modern times, spiritual teachings of both East and West are finding a common link with science. The world is infinite, whether seen from the viewpoint of mathematics or spirituality. Just as an elegant mathematical equation can represent the limitless diversity, creativity and beauty of nature (e.g., the equation that defines the Mandelbrot set), so can keys to the mysteries of space, time and number be found veiled within the Kabbalah.

Debates continue regarding the works of Kabbalah as they relate to the functioning of matter and energy within physics. The connections are evident with a closer look. For instance, when viewed through a Kabbalistic lens, the Big Bang of special and general relativity become the tzimtzum. This blueprint of creation that lives within the poetry and metaphor of Kabbalah contains the key to bridging the macrocosm of special and general relativity with the microcosm of quantum, chaos and string theories.

The many parallels it shares with quantum, chaos and string theories make traditional Kabbalah an exceptional focal point when considering a unifying equation of creation and healing. Originally, electricity and magnetism were considered to be two separate forces, but James Clerk Maxwell's 1873 treatise revealed them to be one: electromagnetism.

As will be explored in greater detail throughout this book, it is not that science, metaphysics, theology or Kabbalah need to change in order to coincide. Rather, it is our consciousness that needs to shift and open in order to grasp the unity within all of these teachings.

Kabbalah is far older than our modern science and, from an ancient perspective, predates even Abrahamic tradition. As a therapeutic tool that utilizes the Kabbalah as its framework, KST is based on the evolution of a healing principal inherent in the very echo of our cells. Kabbalah has traditionally evolved with humanity. The evolution of scientific thought only now touches upon this part of our being and nature, albeit in a deeply profound way.

In order to grasp the concept that Kabbalah is for all, not just man, let us briefly explore the Kabbalistic and KST's definition of Adam.

According to the original Hebrew, Adam was initially both man and woman—an androgynous being. Only later was Adam split into two. Thus, Eve was not taken from the subordinate rib.

Rather, the Hebrew word that was later interpreted as 'rib' also means 'side.' The predominant masculine component located in Adam and the feminine in Eve. Since then, man continues to possess latent femininity, and woman, latent masculinity. This masculine-feminine duality encompasses all of creation yet is united as the whole that is the original Adam. They are beyond the physical world and worlds of dualistic creation.

In the Kabbalistic tradition, an individual's feminine component is more prophetic, prescient, and gifted in spiritual skills. The presence that envelops the prophet or mystic is called the feminine Shechinah (indwelling). The masculine principle tends to relate more to action, expansive movement and giving. Again, these tendencies are not absolutes, as both the latent and apparent aspects of both exist in all dualistic creation.

These dualistic aspects are explored in the following chapters as a part of tzimtzum, sephirot, esoteric anatomy and olamot worlds. They are attributes of a dynamic system for healing within the context of KST.

CHAPTER 3

Sephirot

THE SEPHIROT ARE THE BUILDING BLOCKS OF CREATION. They constitute the framework for everything around us, including the olamot worlds. They also make up everything within us, including our bodies which carry us throughout life. These energy centers act as a bridge between creation and the infinite and provide the vehicle for the desire and expression of physical creation. The sephirot are the first elements of plurality and they exist in all things from the largest olamot worlds to the smallest of quarks or strings.

By learning about the sephirot and working with them on a conscious level, we can help to heal the world, one person at a time.

It takes ten sephirot to make up one building block of creation. Those ten sephirot are connected by twenty-two pathways. Whenever this configuration exists it is called a Tree of Life (ToL). This name implies that each time a ToL is present, so is life.

The top three sephirot are named Keter, Chochmah and Binah. They constitute the intellectual faculties of creation. The six that follow are called Chesed, Gevurah, Tipheret, Netzach, Hod and Yesod. They make up the emotional attributes of creation. The last sephirah is called Malchut which makes up the physical expression of creation.

When we perform KST sessions, we begin working with the sephirot from Malchut and move toward Keter, below to above; rather than from Keter to Malchut, above to below. That way, we are climbing up the ToL rather than descending, helping bring our subject to their highest potential in healing and in life. Each individual sephirah will be covered in greater detail in the chapters to come.

Since the sephirot that make up the building blocks of our body are the same building blocks that make up all of creation, it can be said that the human form is a reflection of the infinite, as is everything else. In this way, we are not *the* center of the infinite universe; rather, we are observing from the viewpoint of *a* center of the universe, one of an infinite number. Integrating this awareness can help us be empowered as individuals and as a part of a greater whole.

This image of a human includes all images, all included within.[5]
— Daniel C. Matt, *The Zohar*

During a KST session, by connecting with the sephirot within ourselves, we can be as a bridge to the infinite healing source of the ohrim (universal healing light). We can connect with the unconditional, pure intention of healing while allowing the ohrim to flow through the sephirot of the client we are working on. We remain neutral during our practice. The healing flow of the ohrim is given a greater opportunity to aid the sephirot of the client without interference from our personal desires and judgments, which are limited by earthly perspective.

The sephirot of the client interacts with the ohrim to aid the client in accessing their highest good and aid the body in healing itself. All we need to do is consciously connect with this process. By doing so we allow the healing energy of the ohrim to flow.

EVOLUTION OF THE SEPHIROT

BEFORE THE SEPHIROT CAME TO BE there was only Ein Sof, the infinite. There was no differentiation whatsoever, just creation before it was created. That was the most absolute unity imaginable. Then creation came into being through the desire of Ein Sof. Part of this creation included duality. Only with duality could the sephirot begin to be defined and the plurality of our existence begin.

Yet, within this plurality, Ein Sof still exists as both the plurality and the absolute unity within. It is only our limited state of consciousness that prevents us from experiencing the truth of this. Ironically, this limitation is valuable because it allows us to have our experience of life as an individual. This personal state of consciousness is what allows us to have free will. Without it, our sense of self would be nullified in a state of oneness with creation and the infinite beyond.

The balance we seek as healers is to maintain our individual state of consciousness while integrating the awareness of unity without getting lost in it. Within the context of life, achieving this balance allows for the greatest freedom of knowledge, free will and personal healing expression.

Traditional Kabbalah says the creation of the sephirot began when the will of Ein Sof, the infinite, contracted to its centermost point and withdrew to the sides surrounding that point. This created a space where existence could begin. Prior to this contraction, the light was omnipresent and there was not room for anything but It.

This process is called tzimtzum. Prior to this, there was no center or space in the literal physical sense. This description relates what occurred in a way that is grasped by our psyche so that we can begin the journey to greater understanding of what is meant by infinite.

Once a space was made, there was room for creation to exist. A single ray of light, called the kav, was allowed to penetrate space. As this process of tzimtzum unfolded, the kav's light was separated into ten different layers, or spheres, much as light is refracted into a rainbow of colors as it passes through a prism. The term *attenuation* describes the decreasing intensity of a sound or light wave as it passes through a medium. As the kav penetrated space, its light was also attenuated. Through this process of separation and attenuation, the light became what we call the olamot worlds and the sephirot.

With the emergence of the first sephirah, the process downward continued. Out of the first Sephirah of Keter the others manifested.

The higher one containing the power of the others and serving as their cause and source. Though we speak of ten different sephirot, bearing different names, we must consider them (as stated above) a unity, for they are contained one in the other and all are contained in Ein Sof.

Ten Sefirot of Nothingness

Their measure is ten
which have no end
A depth of beginning
A depth of end
A depth of good
A depth of evil
A depth of above
A depth of below
A depth of East
A depth of West
A depth of North
A depth of South
The singular Master
G-d faithful King
dominates over them all
from His holy dwelling
until eternity of eternities.[6]
—Ayreh Kaplan, *Sefer Yetzirah*

This above excerpt from the *Sefer Yetzirah* describes the sephirot in one of their multitude of aspects. As a whole, the sephirot are considered beyond human experience; but describing aspects of them makes the knowledge they offer accessible.

The directions listed above relate to the orientation of the sephirot in time and space. They correspond to our experience of axis (teli), as well as space and time (galgal). Teli represents the axis around which the universe revolves and where the physical and spiritual meet. Galgal represents the celestial sphere and the experience of time.

Referring back to the illustration of the ToL (Ten Sephirot), note that the final vessel of Malchut reflects the light of the other sephirot and is the "singular" upon which the purpose of creation is achieved.

The sephirot are a dynamic chain for healing, knowledge, enlightenment, self-exploration and health. This chain provides a structure for our known universe in much the way that DNA provides a structure for our human physical form. The sephirot are the basis for every particle, every star, every person, plant and grain of sand that exists. They also provide the framework for the form of Adam Kadmon, or the primordial human.

The sephirot act as a bridge from which Ein Sof participates with life. Ein Sof fills and surrounds us and all of creation, while simultaneously being concealed from everything. By studying, contemplating or working with the sephirot as healing instruments, we can begin to get a better grasp of life's truth at this level. In doing so, we allow ourselves to become clear vehicles for the universal healing light of the ohrim for the purposes of *tikkun olam*, a *healing* or *rectification of the world*.

The more we practice bringing the lessons of the sephirot into our conscious being, the more efficient we can become as tools for healing. As a by-product of connecting to the reflection of the sephirot within ourselves, we become more connected to infinity.

Once their general descriptions are learned and felt, the sephirot will begin to make sense as an evolutionary whole that mirrors aspects of life and existence. If viewed as energy or light, they can each be seen as differentiated vibrations of the one source of light.

CONCEPT OF THREE

*...Heaven was created from fire
Earth was created from water
And air from Breath decides between them.*[7]
—Ayreh Kaplan, *Sefer Yetzirah*

THE GEOMETRIC REPRESENTATION OF THE ToL contains many mysteries. One of these mysteries includes the concept of three. There are three primary ways that the ToL can be organized. The first consists of three vertical lines, the second of horizontal lines, and the third is composed of three triads. These are the three groupings that should be considered for reference when working with the ToL.

Following is an illustration which shows a brief introductory summation of the vertical columns, horizontal lines and three triads. These will also be addressed in greater depth and detail in subsequent chapters. As you explore the three methods of organizing the ToL, keep in mind that no matter the perspective from which you are viewing it, the structure of the ToL stays the same. Like the two faces and vase of the famous Rubin's vase paradox, these groupings represent different ways of seeing/looking at the same thing

The first set of three consists of vertical lines or columns. According to this view, Chochmah, Chesed and Netzach make up the right column, the element of water and the masculine principle. Binah, Gevurah and Hod make up the left column, the element of fire and the feminine principle. Keter, Tipheret, Yesod and Malchut make up the central column. Keter is associated with the element of aether. Tipheret and Yesod correspond to the element of air and Malchut to the element of earth. The central column is the balance point between the right and left columns.

The second set consists of three horizontal lines called the three constitutions. The upper line is associated with the element of fire and represented by the Hebrew letter Shin. The middle line is associated with the element of air and represented by the letter Alef. The lower

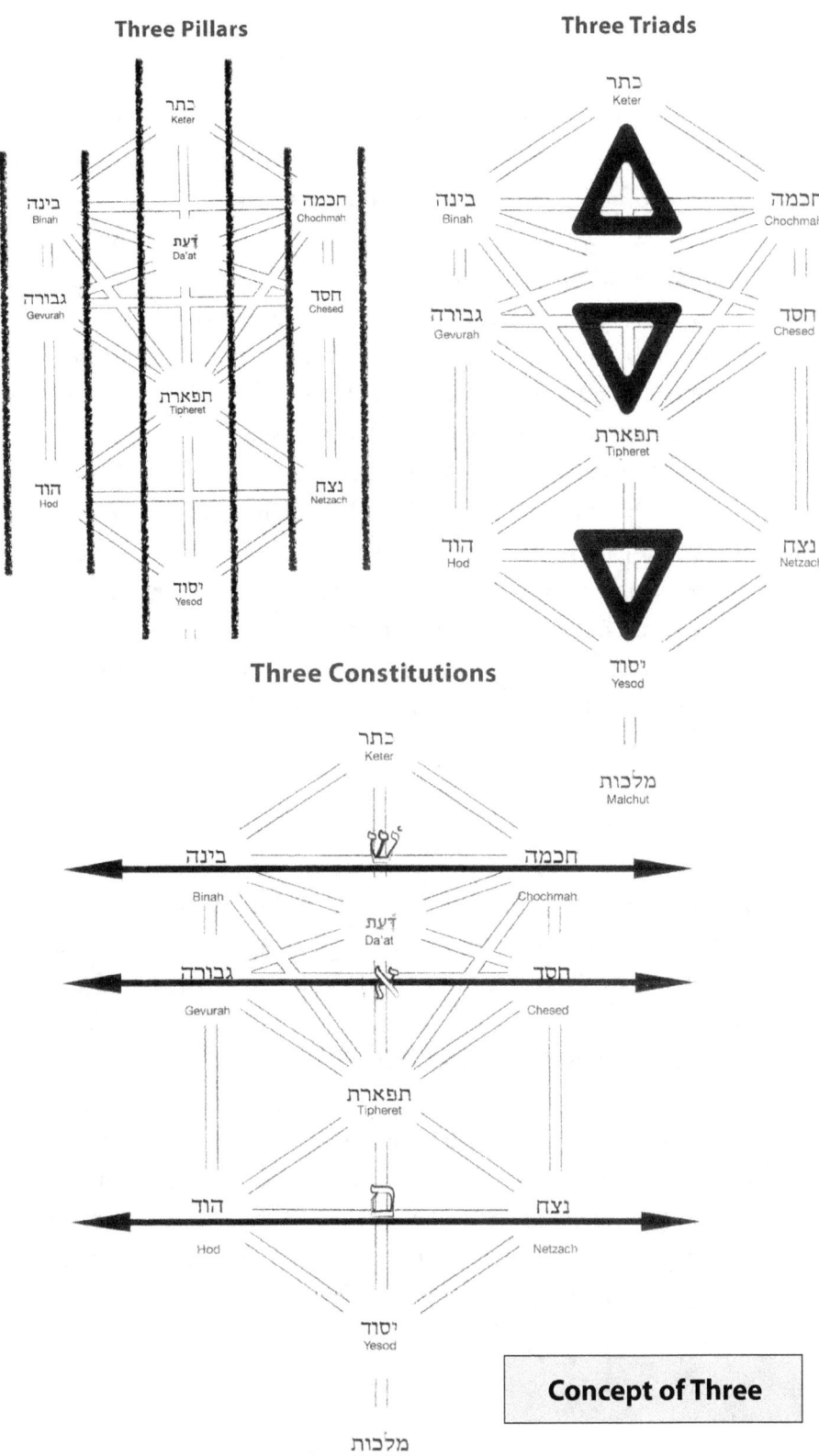

line is associated with the element of water and represented by the letter Mem. They correspond to the three constitutions in KST and the Three Mothers as found in the Sefer Yetzirah.

The third set, that of triads, begins with Keter (crown), then Chochmah (wisdom) and Binah (understanding). These first three are called the Supernal Triad. The second grouping consists of Chesed (loving kindness), Gevurah (severity) and Tipheret (beauty). These three are known as the upper triad of Zeir Anpin. The third triad consists of Netzach (victory), Hod (splendor) and Yesod (foundation), and is referred to as the lower triad of Zeir Anpin.

The last sephirah is Malchut (kingdom), which stands by itself; for it is actually not a separate attribute, but instead represents the harmony of all other sephirot. Malchut acts as a mediator between the sephirot and other worlds. It receives the influences of the sephirot and reflects them to other links in the chain of existence. It is through this mediacy of Malchut that the sephirot are able to act upon the world, hence Malchut's great importance.

SEPHIROT AS ENERGY IN THE BODY

THE SEPHIROT ARE MANY THINGS. In the context of our bodies, the sephirot can be described as spirals of energy, each one a different overall color. They express varied aspects of our emotions, mental state and general well-being within their designated areas of function. In addition to their individual expressions, these sephirot also interact with each other. They serve as conduits for light. From them the universal healing light of the ohrim can flow into the body and aid us in achieving optimal wellness. Studying and working with them helps clear the environment and our subtle bodies of energy that need to be transformed or released. Connecting with the sephirot as the energy centers of our body is the start of a deep and varied journey into the meaning of life.

Ten Sefirot of Nothingness
Their vision is like the 'appearance of lightning'
Their limit has no end [8]

— Ayreh Kaplan, *Sefer Yetzirah*

The above quote from the *Sefer Yetzirah* speaks, seemingly paradoxically, about the nature of the sephirot. How can the sephirot be *of nothingness*, yet be the building blocks for everything? The answer lies in both the enigmatically and the all-encompassing nature of infinity. These answers are all around us, including in new areas of physics such as quantum physics, quantum biology, chaos and string theory. Within these fields of science, it becomes apparent that matter is composed of 99% space. And the closer scientists are able to view that 1% of matter, the more obvious it becomes that even this small percentage of matter is energy as well. When energy vibrates at a slow enough frequency it appears solid to us since our own physical bodies are operating at the same slowed frequency.

Our physical universe consists of different rates and concentrations of energy. Physics postulates that vibration translates into energy; the higher the frequency, the greater the energy and the lower the frequency the lower the energy. Einstein has shown that energy translates to matter as $E=mc^2$. The speed of light, at 300,000 meters per second, became the exchange rate by which these vibrations express as particles of matter (An example of $E=mc^2$, Gordon Goldberg's description of the light from an orange, can be found in chapter seventeen of this book). The sephirot can be said to vibrate at different rates from those of physical light. Within our world, they have their own exchange rate between matter and energy; at the same time, they are beyond the material. They are an evolutionary whole that mirrors aspects of life and existence. If viewed as energy or light, they can be seen as different vibrations of the one source of light where the ohrim is found.

RT: RUAH TECHNIQUE

As the breath wanders, the mind and body become unsteady. When we connect with our breath in stillness, our mind and body are also still.

In order to consciously connect with the sephirot on a level beyond the rudimentary, it is important to connect with ourselves first. We bring our awareness back to ourselves in the eternal now in order to gain a better understanding of the sephirot. RT (Ruah Technique) is a way to bring ourselves into the elusive here and now by connecting with the breath. It is a suggested exercise prior to performing any of the KST protocols.

Breath as ruah is the life principle in the air that we breathe and the blood that distributes it to the earth within us. Without it we cannot experience physical life. Ruah ignites the breath of life within our cells. When breath departs, the scales of life give way to the weight of death. Ruah is also the stored life force in the food we eat and in all things that we are nourished by. It is a form of radiant energy that is the life essence in all living forms.

Within our body ruah is absorbed as air by the fire of the blood stream and mingles to become the vital conveyor of life to our organs and tissues. The heart's four chambers represent the ascent and decent of the pathway of the four elements. We breathe in air as oxygen. Plants expel oxygen as their waste. From our perspective, plants are the upside-down mirror of us; they have their roots below the ground instead of above, and they inhale carbon dioxide as their ruah and expel oxygen as long as they are alive. The life force of ruah exists in all things, and the Malchut of the ToL within each form determines the expression of ruah within that form.

Breath as ruah is the mystery that expresses itself in the central column of the ToL within our bodies. At either vertical extreme of the ToL Keter is consciousness as aether and Malchut is form as earth. The other two sephirot of the central column, Tipheret and Yesod, are air as beauty and foundation, respectively. Within the six sephirot of ZA (Zeir Anpin), Tipheret and Yesod are the breath as ruah is the beauty of our central sun and the gateway of our physical reflection. Breathing techniques such as RT help to balance these sephirot within our bodies and lead us to an awareness of infinite stillness. Within that stillness we can access our purpose and gain awareness on our journey within duality.

Ruah is everywhere; as we breathe, we extract and convert what we need from the air around us, and from the water and foods which we consume. As we become more conscious of how ruah impacts our life and mirrors our reality, we begin to make shifts in food, water and breathing choices. Fresh foods have more ruah than processed foods, pure water has more ruah than contaminated water. Practicing RT provides more ruah for our body than shallow, unconscious breathing.

Ruah is Malchut's nature that helps keep matter pliable. The greater the fluidity and elasticity in an organism the more ruah can be utilized by the tissues of the body. That is the secret of youth. The softness and tenderness of brain, muscle and nerve tissues are good examples. All healthy life is extremely flexible and endowed with energy to play and explore with.

When our bodies become too dense, stiff or resistant, the flow of ruah's currents are impeded. This lack of flow can cause our cells to crystallize and our physical form becomes our tomb instead of a life-giving vehicle. From an impersonal view, even this tomb is ultimately life giving within the Earth that breaks it up and liberates the elements within. The stored elemental energy of our bodies can then be utilized by another ToL to help sustain the creative expression within all of life.

Breathing facilitates life. It is one of our most vital functions. On a physical level, breathing aids us in getting oxygen to the blood, brain and rest of the body. On an energetic level, we connect with the breath to aid in focusing our vital energy and ohrim. Ruah is mostly taken in by the breath. When we perform conscious breathing exercises such as RT we invite ruah into our body consciously. We enhance both the physical body and vital energies through this "science of breath." A practitioner can become clear and connected in a healthy balanced manner.

Ruah is the breath of the ToL in nature. Our physical breath helps to unite our body with our soul. Without the breath of ruah the soul must return to the source from which it came, the agency of that breath of life. The process hasn't changed. Life operates in nature, even though we do not see or understand it in its infinite variety of manifestations. Ruah is the universal breath in nature. Be it gifted as carbon dioxide for plants or oxygen for humans, Ruah sheds its radiance on and through all living things and forms. Such is the relationship of energy within the nature of Malchut.

Where ruah is present in normal amounts, healing and creative expression are supported because Ruah prevents decay. Many issues of imbalance and stagnation within the body are a result of shallow or restricted breathing. This results in excess negative energy.

Life is meant to define light. Because the earth's nature tends to be negative in polarity, and the nature of light tends to be positive in polarity, the goal of RT is to breathe in light. This disperses negative energy in order to help the body restore its balance. This can be done by practicing RT ourselves. If working with others, this technique can be facilitated by us through holding kavana (intention) for another. RT can also be applied when doing more general healing work, such as for the environment or the universe as a whole.

Basic RT Protocol for Individual or Group Practice

1. Sit or stand comfortably.
2. Guide your consciousness to your breath.
3. Relax your jaw.
4. Quiet your mind.
5. Focus on your breath.
6. On the in-hale (which is through the nose), constrict your throat and nasal passages until you hear a wind tunnel-like sound. Continue breathing in with that sound for the full inhalation. Completely fill your lungs and abdomen with your breath.
7. Hold the breath until you need to release it.

8. Produce the same wind tunnel-like sound on the ex-hale (which exits via the mouth). Make sure the ex-hale is longer than the in-hale. Ideally the ex-hale is twice as long. Release all of the breath from your abdomen and lungs.
9. Hold the breath until you need to inhale.
10. Repeat as you inhale.

Perform RT for a few minutes in the morning and a few minutes in the evening preferably just prior to meditation. Do RT prior to conducting a KST session.

RT Protocol for Energy Cleansing

1. Sit or stand comfortably.
2. Relax your jaw.
3. Guide your consciousness to your breath
4. Quiet your mind.
5. Imagine a white light above you. Allow that light to enter through the crown of your head as you slowly inhale via the nose while making the wind tunnel sound.
6. Fill your throat, chest and belly with a conscious breath. Imagine a white light descending with your breath and continuing down your legs and through your feet, connecting with the Earth and continuing further into the depths of the Earth. Imagine the white light transform into gold light.
7. Hold the breath until you need to release it. Exhale through the mouth. Imagine the golden light of the Earth coming up through your feet, your legs, your torso, neck and head. The golden light nurtures you. Allow the golden light to connect and transform into the white light above. Make sure the ex-hale is longer than the in-hale. Ideally the ex-hale is twice as long. Release all of the breath from your abdomen and lungs.
8. Hold until you need to inhale.
9. Repeat as you inhale.

Perform RT for cleansing whenever there is a need to clear the body of an imbalance of energy. The white light is the pure light of the ohrim that brings all that needs to be transformed within us to the Earth. Our negativity is food for the Earth just as our carbon dioxide is the oxygen for a plant. The Earth has the ability to utilize our negativity and transform it into a healing and protective golden light that is gifted to us for health and help. We imagine gold light around us whenever we need protection.

There are many forms of breath exercises that help to consciously connect the worlds of energy to the physical world. Try them all and see what works best. The key is to connect with the breath as a bridge between worlds while living in the ever present now. This is the place where true healing and living begin.

Chapter 4

Malchut

The end is enwedged in the beginning, and the beginning in the end. [9]
—Aryeh Kaplan, *Sefer Yetzirah*

MALCHUT IS THE FARTHEST SEPHIRAH from the highest spiritual realms, yet it is also the closest. It is the ultimate reflection of the intention behind creation. Malchut is the physical world around us and the physical body that contains us. Within this world lies the hidden secrets of unity. Like a pencil refracted in water, the separation of the physical and the spiritual is an illusion.

As individuals, we experience the illusion of being separate from the whole of creation and our lives as separate from others. Since we live in a dualistic world, the reflection we see from Malchut may seem disjointed and separate from the whole of creation. This view is only from our perspective.

Malchut reflects the blueprint of the higher sephirot. The reflection is the illusion we call universe. It is called the World of Asiyah or the physical world.

Unlike the Sephirah of Keter, where there is no differentiation, Malchut is able to contain the whole of Keter's unity while maintaining the illusion of duality. Malchut is the completion of infinity and the initial will which is found in Keter.

Using multifaceted reflections, Malchut gifts us with the spiritual theater of our physical world. Within the physical world, we can make choices freely. Malchut provides us with the opportunity to explore the whole of creation through its different components, including the part that is us.

Malchut acts as the vessel which reflects the remainder of the ToL. There is a ToL in all things. Creation alludes not only to the physical world that we know but also to that which exists beyond our senses or ability to comprehend. The ToL, between Keter and Malchut, is broken down into other individual sephirah. Each sephirah expresses a particular aspect of the whole. Only in Malchut do all of these parts interact. A human being with free will, living in a physical universe, can follow the ultimate purpose of creation which is to have choice.

The first step toward fulfilling our potential in life is to connect with the Malchut of the ToL within us. We do this by gaining an understanding of who we are and how we function in relationship to ourselves and the world. This helps us to make more conscious and constructive decisions in our life.

Malchut is associated with kingship. In this aspect it is associated with dominion over our lives. When in balance, Malchut reflects sovereignty harmoniously. When out of balance it reflects the way in which the outer physical world controls us.

Malchut reflects the other sephirot in the ToL. From the perspective of Malchut, that reflection means "as below so above." This implies that our own actions below impact the sephirot above. Our free will allows us to make choices and act within the reflection from above. Those actions directly impact our avir, or bodies of energy, and the worlds above. Both are inextricably connected.

G-d founded the earth on its base. [10]

— Psalms (104:5)

In traditional Kabbalah, Malchut is counted as the tenth sephirah. This description of creation begins with the spiritual and descends into the physical.

In KST protocols, Malchut is counted as the first sephirot since we are practitioners working as therapists or healers in the physical world, living in a physical body and mind. Our perspective as practitioners begins with the perspective of the physical world. Reality is relative based on where our observations originate.

KST follows traditional Kabbalah by adhering to the idea of the Sephirah of Keter as the first to appear in creation. Yet, Malchut was still the original intention within Keter. So, did Malchut spark the creation of Keter? Or did Keter start the creation of Malchut? The chicken or the egg… in Hebrew, mate-ve-lo-mate, a simultaneous contradiction. Viewing Malchut as the first or the tenth sephirah are both correct. A practitioner is correct counting Malchut as the first sephirah in a KST treatment protocol or counting Malchut as the tenth sephirah in traditional Kabbalah.

When a KST practitioner begins a ToL reading, they usually start with Malchut. This point is at the feet for the front of the body and the lower backside for the back of the body.

We are healers, working with the ToL within the physical world. We honor our incarnation into the physical by ascending the ToL. In this way, Malchut is the vessel for the light of the higher sephirot just as the physical body is the vessel for the soul. This helps create balance in our lives and in our work. By nourishing our personal stability, we are helping to create a base from which to support the abundance, wisdom and health that the universe wants to give to us.

Stability in our lives is usually mirrored by stability in the sephirah of Malchut within the body and mind. Gurumayaji once said, "It is easier to meditate on a balanced checkbook."[11] Stability strengthens the vessel containing our body and mind. We become a vessel achieving our life's purpose. This includes being a vessel for the unconditional healing light of the ohrim. In KST, we act as conduits for the ohrim as opposed to being the ohrim. We can be as this light by acting in accordance with it.

A balanced Malchut allows us to better traverse the expanse of the ToL without breaking our vessel's physical body or mind. It gives us a sense of grounding and balance.

When the physical body is out of balance, Malchut is likely also out of balance. Our entire focus shifts to healing. It is almost impossible to work on manifesting our spiritual purpose in the physical world when our body and mind are not cooperating. With balance, we are free to explore the emotional and spiritual sides of ourselves and the universe. The stronger our vessel becomes, the more the universal healing light of ohrim we can contain and channel to ourselves and others.

The ohrim is plentiful.

It is the vessel that defines how much of this light we can hold and allow to shine in the world.

Next, we embrace the idea of sovereignty over our life. In ancient Israel and Kabbalah, it was said that a king or queen ruled by consent of the governed. Without consent, there existed an imbalance. We use this as a metaphor for our personal life. We are conscious and present. We are grounded in the responsibility and sovereignty that reflects our intentions.

This image of human included all images, all included within. [12]
—Daniel C. Matt, *Zohar*

Malchut reflects the other sephirot. Like actors needing a theatre, the sephirot need a vessel to contain their light. The vessel of Malchut becomes the theater for the other sephirot. Their light is reflected in Malchut in order to enact the events of life.

Malchut grants us, through free will, a sense of individuality. One of our purposes in this universe is to be a witness to creation. Through our interactions with our choices in the theater of creation we can learn about ourselves as individuals. By maintaining our individuality, we have achieved one of the primary purposes of our humanity. We maintain a strong vessel of Malchut, one that fully contains and reflects the ToL. We remain grounded and walk in the spiritual and physical worlds simultaneously.

If we were only the light, we would know the bliss of truth and would follow the will of the light. Angels do not have freedom of choice. They are too close to the light. We are on a path in which we choose and grow until we become co-creators within creation and Ein Sof (without end).

Without Malchut there is no physical experience and the purpose of creation would go unfulfilled.

Malchut relates to the element of earth, and all physical things, such as our body. It influences our health, wealth and our material existence. Once our basic needs are met, Malchut helps us manifest our dreams and purpose.

The KST practitioner reads Malchut at two primary locations. One is on the bottom of the feet, which reflect our lives as a whole. The entire body is mapped out on our feet. The reflection is a manifestation of the reflectiveness of Malchut. Our feet provide a stable contact point to the Earth. Malchut is crucial to our physical existence and spiritual evolution.

The other primary location for Malchut in the body is the anus. It aids us in getting rid of waste that is no longer needed in our lives. We do not connect directly with the anus during KST healing sessions and there is no need to. That could unnecessarily infringe on a client's personal space and break laws in certain jurisdictions. Luckily, Malchut also corresponds to the section of the spine called the coccyx, as well as the coccygeal spinal ganglion and the lower lumbar vertebrae from which this ganglion sprouts. Its connection with the sciatic nerve helps to connect our nervous system to the Earth. Therefore, the feet allow us to release and access energy and information from the Earth into the body.

Malchut typically begins in the low back and hips, a location of support. Then Malchut goes down through the legs and ends at our feet, our connection to the Earth and our final destination. The spinal column provides this connection to the earth, giving us support. This pathway for Malchut provides grounding outlets for us to manifest mind and the body intentions in life.

When our survival is threatened, we may experience fear. Having high levels of fear can be an indication that Malchut is out of balance. Fear counteracts our sense of safety, abundance and calm. KST exercises can help us to face our fears. These tools can direct stabilizing energy toward Malchut.

Not all fear is bad. Short term fear is a primary source of our survival, for example, when running away from predators. But, the ongoing fear, manifested as stress and anxiety, interferes with the healthy functioning of Malchut.

The Hebrew word that is translated into English from the Tanakh as "fear" is actually the word for "awe." This is a healthy fear that helps keep Malchut stable. To have awe is to be in amazement of creation, creator and all that is around and within us. The brimstone crumbles when we understand this simple translation. It can provide the space for moving through life with love rather than with fear.

Many believe that the physical body has no consciousness and only exists to provide us with a vehicle to use and then discard upon death. KSTechnique® allows us to access the more concealed truth within our cells and experiences. The body has its own powerful wisdom to share with us. It is an extension of our consciousness. In accessing a small amount of that understanding, our road to enlightenment and our abilities as healers will unfold exponentially.

Matter is condensed energy. An atomic explosion converts one-millionth of a gram of matter into a hundred million watts of energy. Likewise, we have tremendous spiritual energy in our cells. This energy can be used to create strong vessels for our light. It allows us to integrate universal truths in a grounded way so that we can walk in spiritual worlds without getting lost.

Once we are grounded, the higher sephirot can grant us more freedom as we consciously begin to connect with infinity. We begin to experience the expansiveness of this unification experience. Perhaps, we may become uncomfortable with the constrictions of our daily life. However, these perceived limitations are a construction of a solid bridge to another infinity.

The upper levels of the ToL are not accessible to us in our physical human form. If they were, we would dissolve into the blissful whole of creation without accomplishment in the physical realm. To fulfill our life's purpose here on Earth we must harmoniously ground ourselves as we embrace our limitations, which we learn are not restrictions. Rather, they are vehicles that can take us toward understanding, wisdom and fulfillment.

Out of balance, the physical world and our physical body can feel like forms of bondage. In balance, they can be our greatest strength. As we begin our journey up the ToL, we will understand more about the esoteric levels that find grounding and expression in the magnificent kingdom of Malchut.

GROUNDING

Many meditation techniques only cycle the energy of the upper worlds into the body. Grounding by some of these practices has been labeled as less spiritual or not spiritual at all.

However, grounding *is* spiritual. It is an important step in exploring the mystical realms. Without grounding there can be little manifestation or effect for any cause.

The energy attained from the higher realms should be grounded through its descent down the ToL within the body and into the Earth. Once there, the energy is transformed into a nourishing, golden light. This energy can then be received back into our body from the Earth. Next, it ascends up the ToL within the body and into the higher realms. It is then returned to our body and transformed into a pristine, white energy that enlightens and purifies us. These two energies of gold and white interact with the ToL within us and create a complete circuit of energy. This energy interacts with the rainbow light of the ZA (Zeir Anpin) to help heal, balance, nourish and replenish us.

The Earth is a testing ground for our truth, beliefs, dreams and intentions.

The Earth's negative pole gives us an astounding opportunity to release our own negative energy productively. Our negative energy feeds the earth. Once the Earth processes our negative energy it becomes a golden light. We absorb the golden energy as food for our soul. The energy then ascends through the ToL within us and upward as part of the circuit of life.

It is important to remove the judgment of the word "negative" as bad when speaking about the polarity of the Earth. We previously used an analogy of this as that of a plant that inhales the carbon dioxide that we exhale. It is food for the plant. Once the plant processes the carbon dioxide it releases oxygen as its waste. The oxygen is life sustaining for us. This gas exchange follows a complete circuit from us to the plant and back to us.

Energy distribution is neutral since the cycle is a closed circuit. How we use energy is our choice. For instance, we may feel burdened by negative energy within us and not want to expose anyone else to it. But to hold onto our negative energy is like holding our breath in front of a tree. In doing this, we and the tree would miss out on life-sustaining nourishment! So, let's keep breathing deeply, both in and out. It's vital for us to keep gifting the Earth with any negativity and to be receptive to the golden light that we receive.

Once we learn to circulate energy it is important to ground it. To ground within this circuit we must make dynamic contact within ourselves, with the earth, with its edges and limitations. Become fully aware of the present. That connection is where infinity exists as both reflection and action. When we are present in the here and now we can touch infinity. We can achieve our purpose. We need only open to Malchut, merge with her gravity, and descend deeply into the vehicle of our body.

Beyond the positive and negative poles of our judgment lies the neutral balance of unconditional love.

SHECHINAH

Malchut is often associated with Shechinah, the limitless divine indwelling associated with the skies and presence on the Earth. To access Shechinah is to access the sublime within the mundane. When connecting with this energy, we begin to feel the spiritual existence within the physical. By holding space during a KST healing session we may become aware of the existence of the Shechinah.

Shechinah is often referred to as the feminine aspect of G-d. This g-ddess has been gifted many names and manifestations throughout time. They are all names for different aspects of one reality.

The oldest g-ddess figurine, the g-ddess of Willendorf, was sculpted around 30,000 years ago beginning in the late Paleolithic era of the last Ice Age. With the subsequent Neolithic Age, both agriculture and the g-ddess religions flourished. At those times spirituality was Earth-centered rather than heaven centered. The g-ddess religions were of this world, not otherworldly—body-affirming rather than body-denying—holistic not dualistic. The g-ddess was immanent within all of us, not transcendent. Humanity was viewed as part of nature, death as part of life. Her worship was sensual, celebrating the erotic, embracing all that was alive. The g-ddess was the life force.

KING DAVID

Malchut is both masculine and feminine. For the purposes of KST, we can use the term Malchah, queenship, and Malchut, kingship, interchangeably.

In the biblical Hebrew, both G-d as Elohim and Adam as the first primordial human are written in the plural and contain masculine and feminine grammar. From a higher perspective we are all one. Male and female are polarities within the same truth.

King David is the patriarch associated with Malchut. In traditional Kabbalah, a king or queen would obtain power through the support of the people. Without their consent there would be no legitimate king or queen. This was a benevolent system that represented the divine as sovereign and created us to have choice. King David was a benevolent king who governed with the people's consent. Similarly, we give Malchut consent to support our choice of sovereignty in our life.

QUALITY OF EARTH AS MATTER

The material world may be nothing but illusion —but oh... such an exquisitely well-ordered illusion! [13]
—Anodea Judith

WE SWITCH OUR CONSCIOUSNESS in order to see the spiritual within the mundane. Matter is the ultimate expression of energy. It is one of the highest concentrations of energy possible. Accessing this knowledge is a shortcut to spiritual awareness. Let's consider Einstein's classic equation, $E=mc^2$.

The atomic bomb utilizes fission to produce apocalyptic destruction. Yet the energy released during the atomic bomb's detonation is only three percent of the atom's capacity.

Our Sun utilizes fusion to produce the brilliant yellow glow that warms us. Yet the energy released during the melding of hydrogen into helium in the Suns core is only about ten percent of the atom's capacity.

Imagine that every cell in our being has over thirty times more energy than an atomic blast and ten times more than the sun. That light is an aspect of the spiritual light. We can access it on a conscious level to realize our connection with the vastness of creation. We are smaller than a drop in the universe, yet we have the ability to connect with all of it.

Details for Malchut

Angel: ophanim
Archangel: Raphael, Kaptziel, Sandaephon
Associated Earth element: lead
Body contact points: neck, colon, knees, feet

Chief operating force: gravity
Color: rainbow colors (red, orange, yellow, green, blue, purple, violet) or (white, red, green) or (blue, red, yellow)
Dance movement: floor work, unwinding beginning on floor
Yoga asana: knee to chest, bridge, locus, elephant
Direction: evil (direction away from G-d—not meaning 'bad')
Element: dust-earth
Essential oil: cedar, clary sage, peppermint orange, cedar wood
Finger: left pinky
Food: protein, meat, dairy, anything related to kosher law
Function: grounding, survival, sovereignty, getting rid of waste
Gems: hematite, garnet
G-d's Name: Adonai / Lord
Image: queen, king
Inhabitants: shade of physical world
Location: feet, anus
Malfunction: weight issues, hemorrhoids, constipation, sciatica, degenerative arthritis, knee troubles
Matriarch: Rachel
Meaning: kingship, queenship, sovereignty
Patriarch: King David, Judah. Dan is the lower left leg until below the knee. Naphtali is the foot and heal. Gad and Asher are both the right lower leg and foot.
Planet: Earth
Sense: taste
Spelling of YHVH: YUD HH VV HA (value 52)
Sound: none
Spiritual Experience: Shechinah, experience of the holy guardian angel
Tetragrammaton: Hey
Vice: prejudice, ignorance
Virtue: discernment
Vowel: none
World: Asiyah

Guided Visualization for Malchut

Open to a journey into realms unknown. Ground yourself as you open to exploration into the worlds within—you. Your journey begins here. Your journey begins now. Let all the vibrant colors of the rainbow envelope your senses. Take them in as your breath. Allow them to guide you into your body as the earth. Slow. And let the journey begin.

The earth carries you and has provided you a body to take on this journey. Let your breath take you into your body now. Feel it. Feel the pulsing of your blood, feel the beating of your heart, the moistness in your mouth, the weight of your neck, your pelvis, your knees, your feet, reaching for the ground, connecting with the earth, deep down into the abundance and sustenance of the earth.

Feel your body now. Grounded. Feel its weight, it's mass, it's height. What does the space around it feel like? Speak to your body. What does it say? How does it feel? Are you tired or rested? Hungry or full? Satiated or with desire? How does your body feel about going on this journey? Listen to your body. Listen for the answers. They are there.

It is your own body. It is one of your gifts: a precious vehicle to reflect on your accomplishments and quests. Open to the earth's rich infinity of forms. Feel how its solidity and enormity support you and your path on it.

Take a deep breath into your feet, let it mingle with the energy there. Breathe out and let that life supporting energy flow into the rest of your body. Into your legs, belly, chest, out through your arms, radiating out through your hands, up into your neck, head, flowing out of your nose, up through the top of your head.

With another deep breath, bring your energy back into yourself, into the base of our spine, through your legs and into your feet. Grounded. Solid. Rainbow colors. Earth. Feel your root support, your primal self fully realized. Your journey is just beginning. Your body is on this journey, living on this earth, on this physical plane, it is your grounding, your kingship, your home. You are in the place from which all creation, understanding and action will arise and where all things will return. You are the testing ground of truth.

You are the earth from which all things grow and rest. You are here, you are solid, you are reflective, you are alive.

Contemplation Exercises for Malchut

Following RT:
1. Contemplate a mundane detail in your physical life such as your daily work cycle or washing dishes. Try to see this mundane physical task as a reflection of higher realms. For instance, the water pouring over the dishes becomes flowing, life-sustaining wisdom that is clearing the plate of your life, which can in turn hold another meal to sustain you in order to experience what the universe has in store for you.
2. During your next meal, slow down at least half pace when you are chewing. Really taste the food; feel its texture and sense its smell.
3. While walking, slow down your stride by at least half. Connect with your breath. Feel the air around you and connect with the ground beneath your feel. How do you feel?
4. Choose any daily activity and slow it down by at least half. Slow down and smell that flower!
5. Balance your checkbook.

Chapter 5

Lower Triad

He spoke without knowing what he was speaking—like that radiance of shutting the eye, when the eye ball turns and a person sees concealed light, yet, without seeing. [14]

—Daniel C. Matt, *Zohar*

ZA (Zeir Anpin) translates as, "little face." It is a partzuf, or divine personae, that describes the ineffable qualities of its six Sephirot: Chesed, Gevurah, Tipheret, Netzach, Hod and Yesod. They are often called the emotional attributes that make up the esoteric anatomy of our emotions. These sephirot are located beneath the supernal triad and above Malchut in the mid-section of the ToL.

The upper three sephirot of ZA are Chesed, Gevruah and Tipheret. They are the sephirot of the intellect as a direct reflection of the Supernal Triad above them while remaining interconnected with the three below. Together, Chesed, Gevurah and Tipheret create a balance point within themselves the same way the triad of the three lower Sephirot of Netzach, Hod and Yesod create another balance point. There is much less separation between the two sets of three sephirot in ZA when compared with either the Supernal Triad or Malchut. When intertwined in balance, ZA helps to generate emotional harmony and the ability for us to consciously connect with all creation.

The sephirot of ZA are birthed from the Sephirah of Binah in her aspect as divine mother. They help establish the framework for creation as the emotional material within the physical world. Individually, these sephirot contain qualities that account for key aspects of creation and our experience in it.

ZA is much more accessible to our human sensibilities than the supernal triad that is discussed in Chapter 7, Supernal Triad. The sephirot of ZA are associated with time, space and our emotions. All of these components are how we relate to the world and to each other. They comprise the world we are used to.

The Sephirot of Yesod, Hod and Netzach comprise the lower part of ZA and represent the lower half of the body. Our mind and body intersect at our emotions on a deeply physical level and thus generate our instincts. We are intrinsically connected to our instinctual nature. When in balance, our instincts provide us with extensive and valuable information about ourselves and our environment. This lower triad connects us to the spiritual within the mundane.

Yesod connects us with our sensuality and primal emotions. Netzach and Hod comprise the kidneys on the back of the body where our deepest emotions are held. They are represented in the knees and legs on the front of the body where our emotions can help propel us toward our goals. This triad helps root us into the earth as physical beings living in a material world.

While the upper triad reflects the divine emotional nature of the body, the lower triad reflects our connection with the earth. They are two parts in the same Olamot World of Yetzirah as the partzuf of ZA. When the upper and lower triads are linked and in balance we can access the fullness of our emotions.

The geometric representation of ZA is two interlaced triangles that make up the six pointed star. It represents peace, harmony and unity. This balance occurs when our higher / intellectual and lower / instinctual emotions are in sync. When in balance, they are mirror images of one another.

YESOD

THE SEPHIRAH OF YESOD is the highway for the light of the other sephirot of the ToL and the reflection back to them from Malchut. This is where these emanations of the ToL meet and exchange love, light and meaning. Yesod is the "engine room" of creation since it channels energies directly from Netzach, Hod and Tipheret in order to store and distribute them within Malchut. In this way it is our vitality in the physical world.

Although Malchut is most often associated with the moon, Yesod is also associated with the moon since its domain channels the moon's light as well as the light of the other sephirot into Malchut.

Yesod means foundation. It is located at the base of the ToL just below the rest of the sephirot of ZA and just above the Sephirah of Malchut. As its name suggests, Yesod gives the ToL a stable foundation from which to flourish while providing a direct connection for Malchut. It is the procreative force that descends from the infinite into the finite. It is also associated with the sexual organs. The ideal sexual union would encompass the vision of unifying the higher and lower vibrations of all creation. Yesod is the foundation of the world

Procreation is associated with Yesod. Its flow is responsible for the creative process. It can be related to an infinite array of manifestations such as having babies, transmitting teachings to the world, fertility and union in the world. When in balance, it will help build and heal the world through physical union with the divine.

In the body, Yesod is associated with the genitals where the very act of procreation flows. During the first few weeks of fetal development, the baby's internal and external genital structures are identical, regardless of whether they are going to be a boy or a girl. At this stage the fetus has two sets of sex organs, the Mullerian duct and the Wolffian ducts. The gonads are present in both and will become either ovaries or testicles and the phallus will become a clitoris or a penis. The genital folds will become the labia or the scrotum. Which sex organs develop is based on the male hormone testosterone. Until testosterone has been released or withheld, both male and female genitalia remain the same.

Other organs, such as the fallopian tubes, uterus and upper vagina are also present in both sexes until around twelve weeks. At that stage testosterone becomes present in a fetus destined to be a male, thus making those organs the epididymis, vas deferns, and seminal vesicles in the male. In the female they remain in a similar position to become ovaries, the uterus, cervix, fallopian tubes, and vagina as the labia develops and the phallus becomes a clitoris. In this way Yesod is anatomically represented in the physical body of both male and female.

Yesod represents our physically-based ego consciousness. It is the balance point between Netzach and Hod. This is the chief area of experience for most people. It can either gift us with our limited identity in society or grant us the experience of worlds and universes far beyond our own. It is a gateway. It is our choice to walk through the gate.

It is important to always take care of our physical vessel as associated with this triad so that we have the capacity to carry out our purpose in life. If our physical body is deficient then it needs all of our attention in order to maintain it. When our physical body is healthy we are free to explore other areas of life including the spiritual.

Details for Yesod

Angel: chayot
Archangel: Sandeaphon
Associated Earth element: quartz
Body contact points: shoulders, sides, pelvis, ankles
Chief operating force: weak nuclear force
Color: purple, indigo
Dance movement: camel, snake arms and body, hip circles, hip shimmy
Direction: west
Element: air
Essential oil: ylang ylang, tangerine, jasmine
Finger: left ring finger
Food: seeds, nuts, eggs, seeds
Function: intimacy, generatively, sensuality, sexuality

Gems: amethyst

G-d name: Shaddai (El Chai) (shen, dalet, yud - aleph, lamed / chet, yud) / Living G-d / Almighty

Image: erect male, vulva

Inhabitants: angels

Location: genitals / pelvis

Location on face: nose

Malfunction: impotence

Meaning: foundation

Patriarch: Joseph and Benjamin

Planet: moon

Sense: smell

Sound: oo

Spiritual experience: vision of the machinery of the universe

Tetragrammaton: Vav

World: Yetzirah

Vowel: Shurek

Yoga asana: g-ddess pose, pelvic rock

Guided Visualization for Yesod
Yesod
Foundation
Purple
Air
Interpersonal Connections, Sensuality

Breathe in deeply. Feel the air coming into you... as softness, wisdom, health, breath. Let its nature come into your heart and touch you... move you. Transform you.

Rest. Open. Become a channel for life, a channel for love, a channel for connection, a channel for the universe to express itself. Rest into yourself as you breathe and open.

This purple rose is a gateway for heaven and earth. Allow the earth's multi-colored energy to come up. Let it transform in your pelvis and move you into heaven. Allow the white, opalescent rose light of heaven now to descend into your core, into your pelvis below. Watch it become a bright glimmering purple as it transforms into the earth to become all of the colors of the rainbow.

The light, now healed, transformed, comes back to your pelvis. It's purple rose spins with clarity, healing, calm.

The purple light spins again. It expresses your desires. For what does it desire? In what does it find peace? Allow its dreams to fly upon the wings of transformation, then return to you on wings of blessing, fulfilled beyond your dreams. The foundation for your life that is, for your life that has been and for your life that will become.

Listen deep within.

Every time you touch, you touch your core.

Within each touch is love, awaiting sweet unfoldment.

Release that love upon the winds of the air and breath and reach beyond.

Touch the heart channel inside the ones you love,

And listen to their breath as it journeys back to you... as you breathe in... and out... in... and out...

Ceaseless rhythm of each day is hoping, healing, breathing, feeling.

Let this feeling of connection dance and join the earth to worlds above.

Join yourself with this dance of air and embraced connection.

For within are the seeds of peace awaiting sweet release.

Upon the dual path of these winds of exchange you fly

As deep within you, you cry for blessing

The sweet, sweet call, connecting above to below and below to above.

Contemplation Exercises for Yesod

Following RT:
1. Sit in quiet contemplation. Reflect on who you are. Do you connect with the role that you play in society? How do you identify? Is your role in society a reflection of you? How is it? How is it not? How is this role that you identify with reflected within yourself, society, family, the universe and beyond?
2. Explore your thoughts and feelings around your sexuality and sensuality. Are they connected in your life? Embrace your sexuality exactly as it is. Begin to heal any areas that are blocked by using such statements as, "I release the pain of my abuse and allow health, light, safety and love to fill the space." Clear any areas of judgment in this area by utilizing statements such as, "I release any and all judgment about this situation and ask that it be transformed into tolerance and compassion for myself."
3. For severe abuse issues it is helpful to seek professional guidance as well. We can all benefit from the support of others from time to time. It is what helps create a supportive community.

HOD

You are clothed in splendor and majesty. [15]

—Psalms (104:1)

HOD MEANS SPLENDOR. This sephirah continues our journey into our individual personality as subconscious intellect. Hod represents true humility. It contains a submissive or subduing quality in its receptivity to Netzach's outpouring. Prayer is associated with Hod since, when we pray, we subdue ourselves to a greater force.

Hod is the receiver of the unrestricted instincts of Netzach. Hod is then able to translate those instincts into communicable media, making Hod a key by which we access the flow of mystery from Netzach. The information is then forwarded to the Sephirot of Yesod. This filtered information helps transform unconscious or symbolic mysteries into conscious understanding.

Where Netzach reaches out to another, Hod creates space for another. This space allows room for us to be fully present in a relationship. Its action is in listening or walking in another's shoes. It carries the presence of empathy.

A story says that when Moses died the people cried but when Aaron, his brother, died everyone cried. This is because Moses embodied both serenity and compassion, whereas Aaron embodied only compassion. He only saw the good in people and events. As an extreme example: when his two sons died, he did not cry and was able to see that they had died so as to incarnate into a much greater life. In order to connect with this type of prophecy we must practice seeing the good in all situations. That will help open the door to greater awareness of prophetic understanding.

Another practice that will help heal Hod is to restrict reactivity. For instance, if there is a difficult situation do not be reactive. See the good in the situation. Find the pleasure in it and only then make a decision. It might be the same decision you would have made while being reactive but the energy of Hod will be stabilized. The more you practice seeing the good in people and situations and are not reactive, the more you will stabilize the energy of Hod and the greater clarity you can achieve.

We gain many gifts from healing Hod. They include not repeating the same life lesson and healing a karmic wound that would result in a physical injury. It's a healing across time and space.

In the usual anatomy of the ToL, the energy of ZA (Chesed through Hod) is funneled through Yesod in order to reach Malchut. There is an exception in the case of true prophecy—the energy of Netzach and Hod descend to and ascend from the earth, Shechinah and Malchut directly.

The two cherubs that are depicted on the ark of the covenant represent the Sephirot of Hod and Netzach. To meditate upon their images helps balance the energy of these sephirot. Our westernized depiction of cherubs as plumb little winged babies does not resemble the cherubs of traditional lore. They had a ferocious and powerful winged presence.

The later depiction of the two-winged lions resembled the original. The definition of ZA as "small face" was likely connected to our modern-day cherubs and from there the rest of the body became small and cute. If you prefer the plump babies with fluffy wings perhaps it is what your energy needs to heal Hod and Netzach within you. Only you will know for sure.

Prophecy was prevalent during the time of the temples but not today. Today, we should be careful about people who suggest that they are prophets as it is a rare occurrence. Healers in the higher levels of KST are trained to come close to this level of connection for the purpose of healing. Even then, if connecting is not done entirely for the purpose of healing it can be a tricky road.

Who would not like to know the future? But, how do we know if what we experience is true prophecy? Only we will know for sure. A general rule is if it feels like there is no question about its truth then it is likely prophetic. It has to be as clear as if asking whether or not the chair we are sitting in is real. If there is any question to what a prophecy has divulged then the answer might overlap a prophetic occurrence but it may not be true prophecy. Or, worse yet, it may not be prophecy at all and can lead us down a tangential path or way of thinking.

We are on the path we are supposed to be on. We do not need prophetic insight to be present and do what is in front of us. By taking care of what is present in life we will continue to progress. That is what is needed if we are to grow. The energy of Hod is the awareness of the here and now and being present with who we are in each moment. To help heal Hod practice seeing the purpose and goodness in all that is happening in our infinite here and now.

Details for Hod

Angel: chayot
Archangel: Tzadkiel
Associated Earth element: mercury
Body contact points: kidneys, sides, legs / forehead, solar plexus, thighs

Chief operating force: electromagnetism
Color: orange
Dance movement: up and down maya, hip lifts with emphasis on the down curve
Direction: down
Element: fire
Essential oil: sandalwood, mandarin
Finger: left middle finger
Foods: parsley, white meats, legumes, radish
Function: Intellectual functioning and consciousness, "mind," external personality.
Gems: carnelian
G-d's Name: Elohim Tzevaot / G-d of hosts
Image: hermaphrodite, true duality and polarity in one form
Inhabitant: angels
Location: left foot, left leg, left knee, left kidney
Location on face: nose
Malfunction: disconnection from emotions
Meaning: splendor
Patriarch: Aaron and Zebulun
Planet: Mercury
Sense: smell
Sound: U
Spelling YHVH: YUD HH VAV HA (value 45)
Spiritual experience: vision of surrender
Tetragrammaton: Vav
World: Yetzirah
Vice: falsity
Virtue: truth
Vowel: Kibutz
Yoga asana: warrior I, II and III with left knee out. Standing head to knee with left leg out, tree standing on left leg if attempting to connect with the earth or standing on the right leg if attempting to focus on ZA.

Guided Visualization for Hod

Hod

Splendor

Orange

Fire

Consciousness. Individual Personality. Empathy.

Take a deep breath into your left side. How does it feel there? Gently, slowly, let that energy connect with the base of your spine, let it mingle with the energy there, let it ignite with a gentle fire that warms your kidneys and sides. Be at peace.

Take another deep breath and bring your awareness back into your left side. How does it feel? Gently... slowly, let that energy re-connect with the base of you spine. Let it mingle with the energy there. Breathe out and let that life supporting fire warm and radiate into the rest of your body, into your belly, chest, out through your arms, radiating out through you hands, into your legs, feet, coming to rest in your knees... then back into the sides of your body. Rest... Warmth...

With another deep breath, bring your energy back into yourself, into your sides, into your kidneys. Into your knees.

Hod. The orange rose of life spins, bring your life to a place you can truly see, feel, know as yourself. Know that part of yourself that embraces another, listens to another, wants for another as yourself. Imagine someone close to you... what is happening with them in your life now? Imagine them... listen to them... what are they saying to you? Embrace it... hear it... know it... now gently, slowly, become them... you are the other... look through their eyes... look back at yourself... what do you see? What does it feel like to walk in the others footsteps? Gently, slowly, release them... go back into yourself... to the self that was speaking to the other. Feel the closeness... feel the warmth between you.

Speak to your body. What does it say? How does it feel? Listen to your body. Listen for the answers. They are there. It is your own body...

it is one of your gifts. To listen is to hear your instincts coming to your consciousness, to know them and to cradle them in yourself as yourself.

To listen is to hear the world around you: it's birds and its people, its fire, water and air. Watch that fire as is burns into your past, burns into your future... burns into the present. Feel it's warmth now. Creating a personal knowing, conscious self that is you, that is aware of another, that is aware of it's true self.

You feel empathy for yourself and the world around you. Feel it... know it... be it... You are defined and you are known. Awaken. Open to the world that is you.

Watch the orange rose spin in its compassionate empathy. Watch the prophetic orange rose spin as it offers you its knowing of the world around you.

Contemplation Exercises for Hod

Following RT:
1. Pick an aspect of your life that you would like to receive guidance for. Express this desire as a verbal request, either internally or externally. Think about the words you have chosen. What is their meaning to you? Imagine your body connecting with the Earth's energy—flowing back and forth. Put your ego aside and listen for the answers. Do the words express your kavana? Contemplate them. Then release them as you take a deep breath. How do you feel?
2. Think of a person or situation you are unhappy with. Something or someone you really do not like. Now, contemplate the good in that person or situation. Release them to a better place in your mind's eye.
3. Recall a misunderstanding you experienced. Reflect on what part you may have played in the situation. Next time you are in a conversation, really listen. Then mirror back to them what they

said and ask if that is what they meant. Ask yourself if listening in this way helped to prevent misinterpretation. How did it feel to focus completely on what another person was saying?
4. Meditate on the image of two cherubs facing each other. Allow your own thoughts to subside as the cherubs surround you. Relax into the wisdom and truth that abounds and comes up.

NETZACH

Thighs, joined with two lights–two real lights! Thighs and two kidneys all depend on one place, where all anointing and all oil of the bod gathers, and from there all that anointing is emitted to a place called Yesod olam, Foundation of the world-foundation of the place called world. Who are they? Netsah and Hod.[16]

—Daniel C. Matt, *Zohar*

NETZACH MEANS VICTORY AND ENDURANCE. This sephirah begins our journey into our subconsciousness. Netzach is closer to the subconscious than Hod but it's not strictly subconscious since it is part of the lower emotions. Netzach is rooted higher than all of the emotions but manifests lower on the ToL.

This is where we connect with creation on a primal level. Our instincts and emotions are a direct guide to how we feel about others, our environment and our experiences. It's when we have a sense of a person before we get to know them personally or feeling aware of a place before getting there.

Netzach impacts our sensitivity and creative expression on an unconscious level. More than eighty-five percent of our behaviors and thoughts are subconscious or unconscious processes. We are impacted by this overflowing consciousness yet not aware of it. Within Netzach lies our primordial truth, all artistry, passion and the emotions that makes our life experience feel worthwhile.

The relationship between Netzach and Hod is intertwined. It makes these two sephirot much more interdependent than other sephirot on the other horizontal planes of the ToL.

To connect with our overflowing instinctual nature is to connect with the bliss of life. Netzach is to the soul as Hod is to the mind. Where Netzach is time, Hod is space. Where Netzach contains our unrestricted desire to reach out to another, Hod helps bring that reach into a healthy balance by creating the space that allows another to be present.

The prophets of ancient times were able to have visions by connecting with Netzach and Hod. During the two-hundred years between the first and second temple, our ability to connect with Hod and Netzach were damaged causing a lessening and then a ceasing of prophecy. As a result, accessing the flow of positivity within our subconscious instinctual nature feels insurmountable. But, with practice it is possible and well worth the effort.

Judgment can take a variety of forms. It is our own personal and, most often, negative critique of events, persons, places or things. By applying our personal judgment as to why a certain thing is the way it is or why someone is bad for doing something, we are further damaging the flowing nature of Netzach. It is one thing to have divine judgment as discussed in the section on Gevurah. But, with Netzach the lesson revolves around our personal judgment on a more critical and mundane level.

Our limited human consciousness does not execute judgment on its own. We are only capable of seeing parts of a much greater whole. Without seeing the larger picture how can we possibly know the truth of a thing? To practice getting beyond our critical judgment helps rectify our personal connection with prophetic vision and rectify the damage that was done to Hod and Netzach.

Healing Netzach aids us in being clear vessels for the ohrim. We gain the depth of the six dimensions of ZA in our healing practice. When we are in balance, these channels provide a stable and profound flow for the emanation of ohrim. It is then reflected back to us in a harmonious and stable way. This cycle repeats and helps us continue our climb of the rungs of the ToL. The higher we ascend the ToL the higher our frequency becomes and the more we attract energy of yet higher frequencies. It is the 'like attracts like' scenario. We climb the ToL in balance so as not to falter.

Recall the example of the power plant and the cell phone, in which the power plant is Ein Sof and the cell phone is our soul. What would happen if we plugged our cell phone directly into the power plant? It would be annihilated! Much the same way, being exposed to the Ein Sof directly while in the limited physical body would result in its annihilation. The power from the power plant needs to go through many smaller modes of structure and wiring before it can find the location in an outlet in our home that we can put yet another wire into and then plug that safely into our phone. The more we practice being a clear channel for healing the stronger our vessel will become and the more energy it can hold. The same way, the higher the frequency we are able to contain, the higher the frequency we can attract to ourselves.

Moses, the patriarch associated with the Sephirot of Netzach, climbed all 50 gates to Binah. By calling on that energy we can attain the highest levels possible within our physical human consciousness. As explained in the previous description of Hod, this practice should not be taken lightly. Since these two prophetic sephirot were damaged during the destruction of the first and second temples, it is important to build a strong and positive bridge with them as you climb the ToL.

It is said that the higher we go the farther we can fall. This is very true with all the sephirot but it is especially true of Netzach. Let's say you attain the second rung in the ToL and then you fall. The level you can fall to is not the level you began with. Since you climbed two rungs that also means you can fall two rungs further down than you began with. Likewise, the further you fall the further up you can go… but this is a much messier and more time-consuming way to go.

Those who choose to descend the ToL prior to going up have the unfortunate possibility of not going up in this life time or many more. Just don't do it if you don't have to! Asking for guidance as you climb the ToL is the best way to enjoy the journey and provide sustenance for yourself, those around you and the universe as a whole. Like a parent guiding a child, we ask for help from those that have gone before us.

Details for Netzach

Angel: chayot
Archangel: Haneh or Auriel—grace of G-d or face of the divine angel
Associated Earth element: copper
Body contact points: chest, pelvis, feet / kidneys, sides, legs
Chief operating force: strong nuclear force
Color: green
Dance movement: up and down maya, hip lifts with emphasis on up, shimmy with bend knees
Direction: up
Element: water
Essential oil: Lavender, pine, spruce
Finger: right pinky
Foods: fish, broccoli, kayle, peas, potatoes, zucchini
Function: nature, subconscious, instincts
Gems: emerald, peridot, orange amber
G-d's Name: Adonoy Tzevaot / Lord of Hosts
Image: rose, beautiful naked woman, lamp of awareness
Inhabitant: angels
Location: right kidney, right knee, right leg, right foot
Location on face: nose
Planet: Venus
Malfunction: psychosis
Meaning: victory / thanksgiving
Patriarch: Moses and Issachar
Sense: smell
Sound: ee
Spelling of YHVH: YUD HA VAV HA (value 45)
Spiritual experience: vision of beauty triumphant

Tetragrammaton: Vav
World: Yetzirah
Vice: unchastity
Virtue: unselfishness
Vowel: Chirek
Yoga asana: warrior I, II and III with right knee out, head to knee with right leg out, tree standing on right leg to connect with earth energy or stand on left to connect with ZA

Guided Visualization for Netzach
Netzach
Victory
Green
Water
Unconscious Instinctual Nature

The flow that is Netzach. It's emerald green rose brightens, expands, explores, reaches, reaches. Instincts overflow in this element of water, expanding, constant movement. Open to its flow now.

Be at peace... you are alive... solid... still... yet with each breath there is movement... an ebb, a flow of breath... follow its flow, that part of the stream that glides into the right side of your body. Let the flow of your instinctual nature pool there. a gentle eddy: how does it feel? allow that flowing energy at your right side to connect with the base of your spine... your kidneys... your sides... follow it as it flows into your knees... follow it into the bright green sphere of a rose. A flowing river: tall grass gently swaying. Feel its instinctual waters moving in. Feel them moving out. Sense the change that water brings moment by moment. So slight, yet there. The change, flowing in... flowing out... flowing in... flowing out... this path between worlds, among dimensions, all flow through you in this journey of unconscious change.

Bring your hidden instinctual nature, your unconsciousness, bring it into the sides of your body. Deep, deep into your sides. See the bright emerald green light there. Swirling, pulsating green waters. Rivulets of green light glide down your legs, ebb and flow at your knees, flow back, back up through your thighs, swirling in and out of your kidneys, your sides. The green light moves up through your spine, spreading out through your body, into the universe around you, beneath you, above you, within you, nourishing all of you.

You are the instinctual river of change. Subtle flows of thought, of movement upward, downward, around and through. Find your inner flow and follow it. Your movements, decisions and curiosities are bound within it.

To look into gracious waters is to see a reflection of yourself within yourself. Embrace that reflection. To know yourself is to be free to choose your life in clarity. Allow the instinctual waters movement to gain momentum—removing obstacles, removing tensions. Allow yourself to flow right through and past your obstacles, allow the movement to open you, bring peace to you.

Feel the depths of your water's edge, drift on to your waters depths as you ebb and flow and reach. You taste. Become aware of your body. Sensation.

Your unconscious nature becomes consciousness as it drifts to the sides of your body, emerald green water flows down to your knees, slow swirls around you knees, back up to the sides of your body.

To rest.... To know... to embrace the instinctual self that is you.

Contemplation Exercise for Netzach

Following RT:
1. Sit in quiet contemplation of your own art, be it cooking, painting, making love with your partner, or surrounding yourself with nature's wonders. What feelings, messages or sensations does this impart to you? Listen with your entire being.
2. Imagine yourself sitting near a gently running stream. Relax into the movement of the water. Embrace it as part of you. Expand

your relaxed embrace to include all those you love. Then allow this embrace to include the entire world. See the peaceful Earth within your arms as you look about to see the solar system and beyond. How do you feel?

3. Think of a person you are judging in your life right now. Contemplate why they may be doing what they are doing. Also, try and come up with a scenario as to why they might be doing what they are doing for a positive reason. Internally surround them in the light of the ohrim.

Chapter 6

Upper Triad

That palace is covered with six curtains.[17]
—Daniel C. Matt, *Zohar*

Zeir Anpin: This chapter describes Chesed, Gevurah and Tipheret. These sephirot form the upper triad of ZA (Zeir Anpin), the emotional attributes. They are the higher emotions, or the emotions that are influenced by the intellect. They help generate a connection between the world of ZA and the higher spiritual worlds of the supernal triad. They bring the original intention for our life into stable thought forms which propel us to action. Right action leads to creating our life's purpose. This upper triad is where we write the blueprint for the inspirations we gather in life.

(See illustration on the following page of The Three Triads.)

Each sephirah needs the others to help maintain balance in the world. For instance, what would Chesed's giving be without Gevurah's ability to receive? And what would Gevurah's judgment be without Chesed's sweetness?

Balancing our emotional world holds the key for a full expression and experience of life. Learning the details of the three sephirot that follow will help bring the inspiration of the supernal triad into our life.

Three Triads

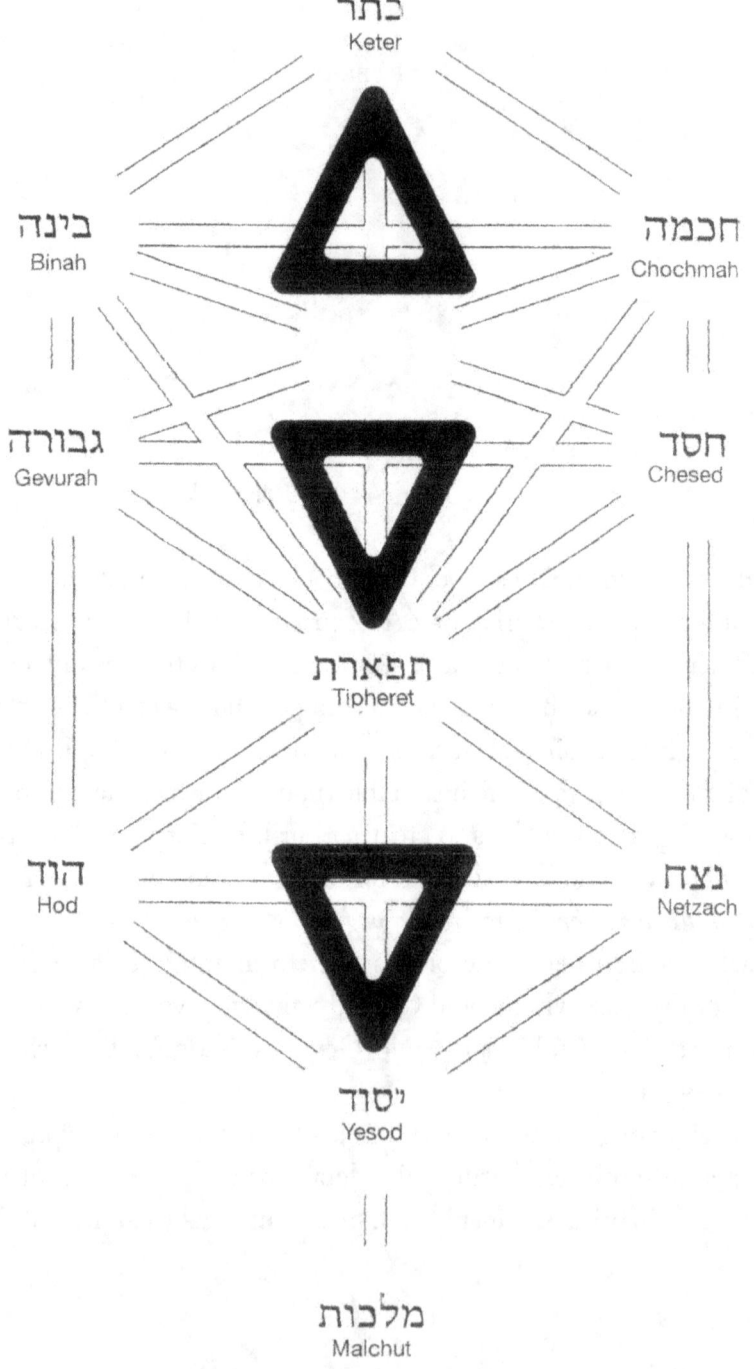

TIPHERET

Tipheret is our central sun that gives tether and grace to the expression of our life.

The Sephirah of Tipheret is a balance point between Gevurah and Chesed. Tipheret provides the counterpoint where both the judgment of Gevurah and the sweetness of Chesed can be harmonious. It is the difference between quantity of life when they are separate and quality of life when they are in balance together. Together they form the rainbow colors.

Tipheret means beauty. It is a powerful energy. This is where we learn to balance opposites. Tipheret is found at the very center of ZA. This position helps balance all of the other sephirot of ZA. It is considered the central point of our emotions and personal identity.

When we connect with Tipheret in our body we can feel it in our solar plexus. It is our central sun that tethers us to ourselves. We can see who we really are at our core. It is where our personal power expresses itself—our stillness in the midst of motion and our silence within the center of sound.

Tipheret is the balance point for all aspects of our nature. This balance point is our eye of the needle that allows us to express the central point of our humanity. If Tipheret is out of balance our thoughts control us, others control us and we are pulled into drama. To find peace we must learn the stillness of Tipheret.

Air is the dominant element of Tipheret. All of the other elements influence Tipheret. This is because Tipheret is sometimes used interchangeably with ZA, which is associated with all elements except for earth.

Tipheret is the tetragrammaton within. It is specifically associated with the Hebrew letter Vav found in the tetragrammaton. The Vav has a gematria or numerical value of six. This represents Tipheret as the one that is central to the additional five sephirot or emotional attributes of ZA.

How do we connect with this energy? We must first balance our shadow with our light and our desire to give with our desire to receive. Tipheret balances the energy of Chesed and Gevurah. When we linger on one side of the ToL we will not be in balance for long. If we reside in the right column of Chesed too long we may be depleted. The left column of Gevurah will eventually make us feel jaded. Chesed is the light and Gevurah is the shadow. As such we require the shadow of Gevurah be balanced with the light of Chesed to be at peace.

Many of us beat ourselves up when we find the negativity hidden in our left column. Don't! Embrace it and bring it into balance as Tipheret. The darkness is what helps define our light. The deeper mystery is that the true nature of darkness is light. Using darkness to create drama in the world is not its nature but rather the misuse of it. Its true nature is light. To misuse it is to seek a false sense of power. As though creation is just an existential toy with which to satiate imbalance. It is hubris. If we are in balance with our shadow, we feel humility, awe, peace and balance.

If we are in denial about our shadow, we are missing a link in connecting with the energy of Tipheret. Don't focus on the shadow too much, just accept it and allow it to transform into an energy that will help to balance and define the light.

Anyone from any background, any religion, any socioeconomic status has the ability to connect with this energy. Keep moving from one column of the ToL (Tree of Life) to the other. Do not stay in one sephirah for too long. Keep moving, experiencing and transforming. Embrace the right column of the ToL, then let go and embrace the left column. Do this until we find balance in the central column.

It is good to see the bad and it is good to see the good. At the highest of levels all is neutral and blissful as long as we don't allow the negativity to create drama. Since negativity is folded light it seeks unfoldment. Drama is an attempt to move the shadow into light when there is resistance to the shadow as light.

It's a paradox to think of positive and negative, dark and light, particle and wave, good and bad, up and down, past and present, as one.

This is the paradox of truth. It is similar to the paradox found within Keter but in Tipheret it is visceral. We directly express our humanity through Tipheret. We do what is right while simultaneously knowing there is a bigger picture of truth. Reaching tipheret consciousness means we are at peace when we are rich and we are at peace when we lose our wealth the next day because we are not enslaved by attachment to money.

With this freedom we find balance and become a vehicle to mediate between the objective physical world and our subjective experience of the world. It is what helps us remain tethered to our core while we explore the outer reaches of consciousness. Tipheret allows us to remain an individual within the bliss of universal consciousness.

Keep pushing and seeking until we know Tipheret is sometimes ZA, other times the chest, above the chest, the nose, the silence, or sun. On the one hand we are the most important thing in this world, on the other we are lower than snail slime. We are both and beyond them both. Once we know who we are no matter what is going on around us we have achieved tipheret consciousness.

Details for Tipheret

Angel: chayot
Archangel: Uriel-light of G-d
Associated Earth element: copper
Body contact points: solar plexus
Chief operating force: weak nuclear force
Color: yellow, green, blue or pink
Dance movement: stomach rolls, locks and chest circles, swaying tree
Direction: east
Element: air
Essential oil: bergamot, lemongrass, lemon
Finger: right ring finger
Foods: grains, especially millet, rye, rice, yellow squash
Function: centering, personal power

Gems: citrine
G-d's Name: YHVH (read Adonai) / Lord
Inhabitants: angels
Image: divine child, eagle, innocent one, mediator balancing cosmic mercy and cosmic severity
Location: torso, solar plexus
Location on face: nose
Malfunction: lack of self esteem
Meaning: beauty
Patriarch: Jacob and Levi
Planet: Sun
Sense: smell
Sound: Oh
Spelling of YHVH: YUD HA VAV HE (value 45)
Spiritual experience: vision of harmony
Tetragrammaton: Vav
Universe: Yetzirah
Vice: directionless
Virtue: devotion to great work
Vowel: Cholem
Yoga asana: bow, woodchopper, wheel barrow, cat, cobra, fish, chest opener.

Guided Visualization for Tipheret

Tipheret
Beauty
Yellow
Air
Personal Power. Still Point

The sound of silence. The sound of silent ever-present graciousness. Peaceful, watching, ever radiant with centered knowing... Observing. Breathe in your sense of knowing. Breathe in and let the flow of breath find its center in you. As you breathe out follow the breath as it radiates throughout all of you. As you breathe in again, find your center and rest.

In that peaceful center you hear this call from above, now coming from within, a call from the very center of you. That vibrant yellow light of stillness. Spectacular... Transcendent... It's your source of personal power... Your personal power that is your core... still point... so clear.

Tepheret. Sephirot of beauty.

Watch the yellow rose spin with its gracious beauty. Element of air. Breathe it in. Watch the healing yellow light spin again—into a thousand suns... into a thousand spaces of breath that connect all other parts of you. Bringing them into—balance. Bringing them into harmony within yourself and the world around you. Bringing them into—a peaceful stillness at the very core of you—the very essence that is your knowing, being, awareness of all that is, awareness of all that you are truly capable of being.

Breathe in that very breath of centeredness. Breathe it into your solar plexus. See the bright yellow light there. Swirling as yellow rose tinged with brilliant rainbow colors... breathe out and let that beautiful light connect with all that is you... connect with all that is beyond. As you breathe—take in your clarity of purpose. Ingest it. Know it... breathe out and know yourself as part of this infinite universe... Know the clarity of the bright, iridescent, shimmering yellow rose of light that is you: connecting you to yourself. Rest. Observe. Be at peace.

Watch this beauty of your thousand suns, see them connect with the beauty of your single moon. Rest in the bliss of connection... of knowing... of observing your centeredness... of observing the universe around you, of observing the beauty that is you... your peaceful knowingness.

Deep in the core of your belly the yellow light spins. The rose expands in light. It's glow illumines the space within you. Glows with the vision of your true self. See it. Go into the space that feels, observes, knows.

How do you feel now in your body? What does the stillness in your center say to you? How do you feel about yourself and your place in this world? The yellow light spins. Rose opens. Caresses.

Contemplation Exercises for Tipheret

Following RT:
1. Bring your conscious awareness to your solar plexus. Find a center of stillness. Watch this center of stillness glow and become a radiant golden light. Rest in its peaceful silence for at least six minutes.
2. Visualize the water element expanding from your right side and moving across your chest to your left side, down your left arm. Then visualize a fiery glow radiating from your left side. Visualize the fire coercing up your left arm, across your chest into your right arm and rising until you are aglow. Now visualize the water element and the fire element combining at your center as they dance between your right and left sides.
3. Observe the heat of the fire warming the water and the water cooling the fire. Allow the warm glow of the water and the fire to expand in a comforting embrace at your core. Let that feeling expand to encompass all of you. Rest in the warmth and find the peace and beauty there as it becomes a yellow sun.
4. Get a piece of paper and make two columns. Write down four of your most negative attributes in the left column. Leave space between each one to have a place to write a bit more about each one.
5. Breathe in your two extremes from number 4. Then write down four of your most positive attributes in the right column. Leave at least two empty lines between each one to have a place to write a bit more each one.
6. Beside each attribute list how it expresses itself in your life. Under that write what you gain from the actions of these attributes. Observe the columns without judgment.
7. These columns are parts of yourself that help you express in this world. Close your eyes and visualize both columns in balance within you. Breathe in your truth. Breathe out imbalance.

GEVURAH

GEVURAH TRANSLATES AS JUDGMENT, POWER OR STRENGTH. Work with this sephirah to focus on boundaries, restrictions, and transformations. Gevurah is the place where both darkness and light reside. In the sense of mate-ve-lo-mate, Gevurah's judgment is both good and bad, depending on the perspective and timing.

To judge a situation based on slander is Gevurah out of balance. To assess a potential personal risk and make decisions that would ameliorate that risk is Gevurah in balance. A good litmus test to notice if we are in or out of balance with Gevurah when it comes to judgment is to ask if our judgment creates separation from the light. Separation indicates an imbalance of judgment. Bringing light to a situation represents a balanced Gevurah.

Pressure is also Gevurah. This is different than the pressure felt from the Sephirah of Keter. Gevurah can take the form of trying to force someone to change. This will likely be a misuse of judgment as that tends to effect separation. Embodying the light is usually enough to encourage change in others. We need to act in accordance with the change we desire. Others will see our actions and be influenced to act accordingly if they are ready to do so. It is not up to us if someone does change. It is up to us to remain non-judgmental about what others do.

The power of gevurah consciousness is knowing that any challenge we face is there to help us fulfill our potential. Like a hermit crab, painful judgment breaks us out of our comfort zone of a shell. It forces us outside. Though our original home was comfortable, it had become too small for the additional light we need to grow. The painful judgment breaks our shell. Our home expands in size. Though our original shell contained light, Gevurah provides even more light in the larger shell.

Surrendering to the judgment of Gevurah shows us our deepest truths. We face the fire of transformation. This intense pressure is reminding us that it is time to embrace our shadow with the light. It's not an easy path but it's worth it. We begin with facing our fears, denial, hurts and lost hopes. When we connect with our shadow, we ask those shadow or hidden parts for their story and listen for the answers. We develop an insight into our sadness, our fears, our hidden hopes and our dreams. If this process becomes too intense to bear alone, we ask for help from a therapist, KST practitioner or other professional.

There are a number of KST exercises that help create a space for such encounters with the shadow and judgment. They provide a safe way to unfold our darkness into light with creative intelligence and social support. By seeking out support, we learn to manage our sadness or fears.

Many other traditions shun, deny or demonize the process of embracing the shadow with the light. That is okay as well. Sometimes we need to take a break from the depths of self-exploration and rest. It is a step wise process. It is not necessarily for everyone in this lifetime. The key is not to demonize, deny or judge others that do this work. To deny the shadow as found in Gevurah gives the darkness false power.

We do not to mistake the shadow for evil. Rather it is a part of us as a reflection of a greater universal truth. The shadows true power comes from its true nature as part of the light.

Maintaining a state of balance with our own light and shadow within Gevurah while holding space for another to heal is power. Bearing witness in a world of shadow and light is in accordance with Gevurah's purpose. That is power. Creating space for the light to heal is power. Holding kavana (good intention) for the world to heal and evolve into enlightenment defines Gevurah's purpose for us as healers.

To know our shadow as black fire on white fire is to be in tune with our true nature as shadow and light. Many ancient traditions say their supernal writings were written with dark fire on light fire as a mirror for this truth.

There is a parable of the seeker who wanted nothing more than to know G-d. Lifetimes were spent in genuine pursuit of this ultimate knowledge. Limitless acts of kindness were accomplished. At last the seeker attained the frequency of the 50th gate of the ToL (Tree of Life). The seeker had climbed the ToL with profound humility and was able to walk through the sacred gate without being annihilated by the light. It was there that the seeker was given the opportunity to request anything they wanted. The seeker said they wanted to know G-d. It was only then that G-d's dark side was revealed as part of the light to the seeker.

The gametria for Gevurah is 216. The gametria of Chesed is 72. If you multiply 72 by three sephirot you get the number 216 that is needed to balance Gevurah. Thus, this truth may be accessed within the gametria of both Gevurah and Chesed even though they are two seemingly diametrically opposed sephirot until they are added with Tipheret between them.

When enlightenment occurs, both polarities of left and right are revealed as one within the center of the ToL. The two polarities grow from the central point the way the limbs of a tree are bound to the trunk.

The left side of the ToL was courageous and strong enough to contain both apparent-light and enfolded-light as darkness, to give us the opportunity to have freedom of choice. If all light was folded in on itself there would be no freedom of choice since we would be crushed. However, the same lack of choice is true if all light was apparent since we would all want to do and be like the light.

By folding parts of the light into shadow on the left side of the ToL, unfolding it on the right and breathing between in the middle, we are given choice. We can choose the left, the right or the middle. We can choose to climb up or descend down. We can choose to be a part or beyond it all. Having some space and time between making these choices and experiencing their effects gives us even greater choice since we do not necessarily connect the cause with the effect.

When the judgment of Gevurah prevails in our life it means that cause and effect are so close we cannot help but connect the two. For instance, as soon as we reach for the cookie jar our mom walks in and yells at us. This limits our freedom of choice to sneak a cookie as we are less likely to continue to reach for the cookie jar while there is screaming in our ears.

There was an experiment done by Walter Mischel in the late 1960s and early 1970s. It was called the Marshmallow Test. In it a child was placed in a room with a marshmallow on a single table. The child was told that they were going to be left alone with the marshmallow and that if they did not eat the marshmallow by the time the experimenter returned the child would receive two marshmallows. Most children ate the marshmallow right away. A few attempted to wait a bit but could not resist the tempting morsel. Only a small percentage made it to receive the ultimate reward of the two marshmallows. As these children were followed throughout life it was found that those with the greatest ability to restrict their desires, by not eating the marshmallow until the researcher returned, were able to do better in school and life compared with the children that ate the marshmallow right away. Being able to restrict our desire, whether it be for a cookie or a marshmallow, is a good way to help balance the energy of Gevurah and find success in life.

The greater our ability to restrict, the greater our capacity to balance the energy of Gevurah in life and within ourselves.

Practicing restriction is key to developing a balanced Gevurah. Restriction includes establishing better personal boundaries and assessing situations before taking action. It means breathing through the rush of desire until it subsides. We must wait until it is the right time to do or receive the energy we want.

When we maintain healthy boundaries, we may not get someone else's energy right away. We may be vulnerable to feeling rejected. To step back before making a decision means not grasping for the rush of jumping in without thought. It risks the possibly losing the source of energy we desire. These are short term concerns. By practicing restriction, we create a stable vessel for even more energy to come into our life. And more stable energy means more blessings.

To ask without preparation is to get burned by the light and fire of Gevurah. This is because when you ask before you are ready to receive you may experience the cost of the request right away. That is Gevurah without the sweetness of Chesed. It's a place where cause and effect are so closely linked in time that there is no wiggle room for easing the judgment of Gevurah. The greater the energy of Gevurah the more we experience judgment at shorter and shorter intervals until we are dragged toward enlightenment kicking and screaming.

Today there is more light available to us than any other time in history. So why are there fewer, if any, true prophets? It is said that back when Kabbalah was originally practiced, the small amount of light that was there was able to be harnessed. People knew how to be vessels to contain the blessings and light of prophecy. Today it is far easier to be shaken off balance or burned up from the additional energy. Practicing such techniques as found in KST, Kabbalah, Ayurveda, Chinese Medicine, Reiki and Polarity means we can harness abundant light. For those whose vessels are not prepared, the experience of an overflow of light can be searing.

Gevurah, as severity belies a deeper truth about our physical world. It is not cruelty so much as the absence of mercy. The merciful hawk who does not eat, soon dies. In this sense Gevurah is "nature red in tooth and claw." This differentiation allows for a greater sense of cosmic order within the physical world. Gevurah does not start fights, wars or conflict. Rather she is the natural cure for imbalance in the world.

Unconditional love is the blend of Chesed with Gevurah.

Details of Gevurah

Angels: chayot
Archangel: Gabriel. Khamael—angel of justice and severity that tests the purity of intents
Associated Earth element: nitrogen, steel, iron
Body contact points: left hands, forehead, solar plexus, thighs

Chief operating force: electromagnetism
Color: red
Dance movement: staccato arm and hand work with emphasis on the left side. Spin to the left.
Direction: north
Element: fire
Essential oil: sage, spearmint, myrrh
Finger: left index finger
Foods: chili peppers
Function: to judge, restrict, define
Gems: ruby, garnet
G-d Name: Elohim Giber, strength and power
Image: warrior in his chariot, ox
Inhabitants: angels
Location: left hand / arm
Malfunction: insanity
Meaning: judgment, severity
Patriarch: Isaac and Simeon.
Planet: Mars
Sense: smell
Sound: Schwa
Spelling of YHVH: YUD HA VAV HA (value 45)
Spiritual experience: vision of power
Tetragrammaton: Vav
Universe: Yetzirah
Vice: cruelty
Virtue: courage
Vowel: Shva
Yoga asana: breath of fire. sun salutation, side to side arm flops, left arm circles

Guided Visualization for Gevurah
Severity

Red

Fire

Boundaries. Discernment. Judgment

A red light spins, sparkles, ignites and glimmers just above. Gevurah, the radiant red rose of fire. It is there. Your personal boundaries burn bright. Your will is strong. Dynamic.

Transform your desire into form.

Feel the cool / warmth of the red light touch the fingers of your left hand. Cool / warm red light covering you hand, entering you left arm. Bring your consciousness into your left arm. Feel the energy there. Allow a warmth to radiate through it. Embrace it as it burns through your chest and down you right arm. Feel the flowing energy, transforming, pulsating, bursting into the flame of transformation. Feel your arms now. How do they feel?

Feel their definition. Their weight, their length, from there you call for movement. The energy ignites into the creative force of fire. Watch as the red rose spins. Imagine your arms reaching out into the world… your fire extending into the universe far beyond where your arms can't even reach. Helping you reach further in order to create and define your desires.

Reaching, grasping, caressing, changing the forms around you, changing your destiny into you true life's spark of purpose. From this spark you invoke fire, the fire of the place between—between you and all, between past and future, between the known and the unknown.

Sparks burst before your eyes. You turn toward their glow and watch as they move, dance and spin about, connecting and igniting all that they touch. A spark touches you, touches something deep within, igniting strength, action, will. Sparks fly about bursting with joy, igniting everything around you, creating other fires… they explode, burn bright… and just as quickly… are gone.

You are lifted, you are so light. Feel your body sway with the rising heat, watch eyes of fire moving within you, expanding, compressing, exploring, expanding and contracting again, ever searing, binding.

Your body now burning, radiating heat and light and strength and will.

Power pulsates through you, above you and below, around and through. Feel this light transforming obstacles within you—transforming them into your desire manifesting before you—all that is within you. Breathe in your life.

Watch the red rose spin. Its light. It's warmth. Let it settle now into your arms, into your left arm. Settling, calming as it gently warms your body now. The bright red fiery rose spins and offers you your destiny. What do you see? How does it feel in your body now? What has been transformed?

Exercises to Balance Gevurah

Following RT:
1. Sit quietly. Search for an area of your life where your boundaries are not strong. Recreate a circumstance in your mind's eye that has occurred or could occur, involving a lack of boundaries. If you are recreating a situation that has occurred but you wish had been different, allow it to be different now by imagining the event differently. Imagine it in a way that honors you and your boundaries. In your imagination, allow your reaction to occur in a way that would facilitate a positive outcome. Likewise, If you are creating a potential scenario in your mind, make sure that your boundaries are secure and facilitate a positive outcome for yourself and those around you.

    Since your mind does not know the difference between external and internal reality, this exercise will help to shift your consciousness, with regard to your boundaries, on a cellular level. Remember the truth of what happened while allowing the alternate visualization to heal you. Be sure to recreate the situation within your mind in a way that empowers and honors you, but does not diminish another.

2. Think of something you are attempting to master. Perform a literal task that brings you closer to mastership of your subject. Do this for a set time each day or each week. See how much you have learned after doing this exercise consistently over an extended period of time. As you progress, remember not to look at the mountain you may be attempting to climb as it may be overwhelming. Rather just focus on attaining your goal one step at a time. Make the journey the goal.

3. Keep a dream journal by your bed. Write down any dreams you had during the night upon waking. As you do this you may become more aware of your dreams. Should this lead to lucid dreaming please find some suggestions on what to do below. These techniques will help to balance the energy of Gevurah:

4. If you are running from something or someone in a dream, turn around and ask why they are chasing you or what they want. If you are falling in your dream try and stay conscious of the dream even after you hit bottom. What do you see? If you have woken up prior to reaching the bottom, see the dream through in your waking imagination. Let your imagination flow and see what is present after the fall. If your imagination is not flowing, choose a scenario of what you would want to see and imagine it.

5. The next time you find yourself in a discussion that is becoming heated or one where you want to pressure someone into your way of thinking, stop. Listen without interjecting. Guide instead of using pressure.

6. Recall an incident, be it large or small, where you had a judgment. Really look at the situation from a higher place. See it in the context of a much larger interplay of life. If it was a judgment of someone else, walk in their shoes for a few moments. If it was a judgment of a situation, what are you judging and why? If there was a personal disagreement, explore your part in it and what you may have learned from it.

CHESED

CHESED MEANS MERCY OR LOVING KINDNESS. It is the sephirah of love as giving. Chesed is sometimes called "cohesive consciousness." It contains all the holy powers and spiritual virtues from which it emanates. Whereas Binah is more the potential of manifestation, Chesed is the blueprint for it, much the same way the etheric field as Zelum Elohim is the blueprint for our physical body.

We experience chesed consciousness on many different levels. Psychologically, Chesed connects us to our collective unconsciousness through the formation of archetypal ideas. Archetypes are universal representations. They act as a bridge between our individual sense of self and the collective unconscious. Both archetypes and the collective unconscious are terms coined by Carl Jung. If we look through this wider lens, these concepts become a type of unification experience with all of humanity. When we bring that experience back into our individual lives through interpretation, they are guides for our life. For instance, archetypes in dreams can tell us what our unconscious mind wants us to be aware of.

Charity, giving, hospitality and overflowing energy are the nature of Chesed. The more we perform actions aligned with Chesed's frequency the more we can expand as loving, peaceful beings of healing and light. In showing generosity, we become more open to receive the blessings of Binah. This may feel counter-intuitive. It is the way of mate-ve-lo-mate. With it, we are able to live in two worlds at once: in the world of giving and in the world of receiving.

When we encounter chesed consciousness, we experience a type of unification experience. There is also a simultaneous understanding of the purpose of creation in-clothed in a feeling of unconditional loving kindness.

These spiritual experiences are often transient, not because we are unworthy, but because we are human. Our free will requires our human form. Were we to exist in chesed consciousness all of the time, we would lose our sense of free will to an overwhelming feeling of bliss.

Many want to give without restriction. Although that is a nice concept, it is not human nature. Once we have given all we have there is nothing more to offer except the desire to give with only the ability to receive. There needs to be balance even in our desire to give within Chesed.

Another aspect of Chesed's character relates to it being the first of the six sephirot to have been birthed by Binah. Part of Chesed's nature as the first born sephirah is to want to be the only sephirah of ZA (Zeir Anpin). In balance, it is the desire to exist as one. Out of balance, the desire is like an only child who wants their parents' full attention at all costs.

Chesed's overall gametria or numerical value is seventy-two which correlates to the entirety of the creative potential. Access the power of seventy-two to be a balanced channel of Chesed.

A way to align ourselves with all of these characteristics as chesed consciousness is to bring opposites together in peace. For instance, if there is a disagreement, step back and focus on the opposing view. Is there is a way to make peace? Chesed consciousness brings alternative ideas harmoniously together as one.

Nurturing characteristics such as peace, mercy, truth and righteousness are attributes to grow toward Chesed. These attributes are the same frequency as Chesed. We surrender and align with the frequency of Chesed by embracing these attributes.

Even when embracing truth there is a need for balance. If you hold to your truth in order to keep what's your's-your's and what's their's-their's, it can create division. To embrace the truth in the frequency of Chesed is to change the consciousness of what's yours is yours to what's mine is yours.

Do not give your things away if it isn't warranted. Develop the ability to become unattached to your physical possessions, setting ownership aside for truth. Feel a sense of truth or righteousness within judgment. Mate-ve-lo-mate helps determine the frequency required to embody Chesed.

Fairness is a shadow. Every time you say that something is not fair and every time you want to live by what is fair, you live within the shadow. It has been said that holding unto your judgments can potentially endanger the community. The traditional question posed is, 'Do you want a speaker of peace of a bringer of peace?' Do you want the mercy of Chesed to decide the truth or the severe judgment of Gevurah to do so?

According to chesed consciousness, a psychotherapist hopes for a day when the entire world would be healed of mental illness. Likewise, a bodyworker would desire that the world be free of stress. We dream of waking every morning to a world of no problems even though we will become unemployed. The ultimate Chesed is when all of us work together to create a society of peace.

Why is Chesed so difficult for most of us to embody? Selfishness is necessary for survival. Children only think of their own needs. They need to do so in order to survive. As children grow, they have the faculties to take care of themselves. Only then can they become empathetic of others' 'needs. Some of us move away from selfishness more completely than others. Moving beyond our selfish desires is to embrace Chesed.

Details for Chesed

Angels: chayot
Archangel: Michael—the righteous of G-d
Associated element: carbon
Body contact points: hands, chest, pelvis, feet
Chief operating force: strong nuclear force
Color: blue
Dance movements: spinning to the right, snake arm and hand work with focus on right
Direction: south
Element: water
Essential oil: lavender, roman chamomile, blue tansy
Finger: right middle finger
Foods: blueberries, lettuce, green salads

Function: law giver
Gems: sapphire, lapis lazuli, turquoise
G-d's Name: El / G-d
Image: crowned king, throne, lion, wand, cube
Inhabitant: angels
Location: right hand / arm
Location on face: nose
Malfunction: lack of love
Meaning: love or greatness
Patriarch: Abraham and Reuben.
Planet: Jupiter
Sense: smell
Sound: Eh
Spelling of YHVH: YUD HA VAV HA (value 45)
Spiritual experience: vision of love
Tetragrammaton: Vav
Universe: Yetzirah
Vice: bigotry, hypocrisy
Virtue: obedience
Vowel: Segol
Yoga asana: sun salutations, right arm circles

Guided Visualization for Chesed
Chesed
Love
Blue
Water
Our desire to give unconditionally

You are safe here. You are safe in the embrace of wisdom's love. Ever giving. Ever loving. Cradled. Quiet. The faint smell of a rose. You are growing. In this peace there is but one truth—the flow of life—the flow of love—the life-giving flow of water.

Allow the blue waters of the rose of love to open, spin and flow forth into all that is you. Allow its scent to flow and fill you with an answer for every dream, every desire.

Open to it now. It is there. In the element of water. So sweet. So clear. Chesed. The sephirah of love.

Be at peace... you are alive... feeling... solid... still... yet with each breath there is movement... an ebb, a flow of breath... follow it into your source... follow it into the bright blue rose. Find it swirling at your right arm. Let its waters undulate until they overflow through your chest... into your left arm... feel the water flow back.... and forth.... back... and forth. Cleansing your heart, nurturing your body.

There is so much water. So much love. It is overflowing. Bring your consciousness into your desire to give the water that is overflowing.

Deep, deep into your journey. See the bright blue light there. Swirling, pulsating blue. Rivulets of blue light glide down your arms, touch your legs, your feet, flow back, back up through your thighs, your pelvis, your torso, your arms. The blue light moves through your spine, nourishing all of you.

You are the river of giving. Subtle flows of thought, of movement upward, downward, around and through. Find your inner flow and follow it. Allow its movement to gain momentum—removing obstacles, removing tension. Flow right through and past them, allow the movement to open you, to bring peace to you. Feel the depths of you as you ebb and flow and reach. You sense and smell the sweetness.

Become aware of your body. Sense it. Let the awareness flow into your arms, your skin. Your waters ebb and flow, nurture, cleanse and heal. You flow with each movement, each yearning. Within each breath you are united. Ecstatic, you merge, complete within yourself. You dance, and rise and fall... and rest.

Watch its healing blue light spin. To your right, the light begins. To your left, it embraces. To the whole of you the light gives unconditionally. Always loving. Always giving.

Its light expands and flows. Its glow illumines the space within you. The space that feels, moves, smells, desires. Take in its fragrance. How do you feel now in your body? What does it say to you? The blue light spins. The rose opens, caressing as it flows. Liquid light. Liquid blue light of a celestial scented rose.

Feel its flowing movement, cascading in, and flowing out. Sense the change occurring at each moment, with each drop as it forms into the flow within you. So slight, yet the flow is there. The change, flowing in, flowing out, flowing in, flowing out.

Embrace the flow. Touch it. Smell it. Feel it crying, yearning, hoping, healing, loving, transforming. Feel it within you, always with you, showing you direction, guidance, the wisdom of your higher self-whispers to you, so wanting you to hear. It calls for your intuition to awaken, your hearth to know truth. A call to memory, for the primal awareness that you are one with all that is around you, one with all that is within you. It is all one. You are as one with the universe.

Contemplation Exercises for Chesed

Following RT:
1. Sit in quiet contemplation. Visualize a pristine, clear blue stream as it flows past you. Its gently crackling water glides over smooth rocks and around patches of grass and trees growing along its banks. The flow of this stream is never hampered by any blocks; it just keeps flowing and moving forth, ever changing, ever flowing.
2. Close your eyes and visualize a time you felt loved. Breathe in that moment. Then, gently raise your arms and embrace yourself as you gently rock back and forth. Internally, tell yourself that you are loved and embraced by the universe.
3. The next time you are about to enter into an argument, stop. Connect with your breath and ask if this argument will bring

separation. If so, try to step back and breathe a calm loving breath. If, in your breath you find that this argument reveals light, then it is okay to act… but this is a rare exception. It is often difficult to tell the difference between bringing the light and just wanting to prove you are right.
4. Perform a water purification ceremony. That can be a peaceful dip in a bath or other body of water while meditating or contemplating your purpose in this world.
5. Study spiritual or uplifting texts between midnight and sunrise.

CHAPTER 7

Supernal Triad

This palace is open—eyes never asleep; gazing constantly, to illumine below from the radiance of that ongoing, that Understanding, concealed Wisdom, is Will of Wills—concealed, treasured away unrevealed, existing and not existing.[18]

—*Zohar,* Translated by Daniel C. Matt

THE WORD SUPERNAL MEANS SKY OR THE HEAVENS and refers to the celestial nature of the three upper sephirot on the ToL: Keter, Chochmah and Binah. Together they represent the supernal triad, three aspects of the same divine essence. They are the intellectual sephirot and function as three components: creative intention, wisdom and understanding.

Keter is the creative intention, the original seed that started the process of creation. Chochmah as wisdom, receives Keter's inspiration. Binah is the channel for the flow of Chochmah's wisdom. Binah imparts wisdom as knowledge to the sephirot of ZA (Zeir Anpin).

By connecting with our own desire to create, contemplate and understand, we are reaching for the supernal triad. We are able to shift our mental perspective and facilitate the change we want. As we experience the upper aspect of our existence, we are able to become co-creators of our life plan. Working with the supernal realm offers us the opportunity to experience the divinity within us. These three sephirot provides a way to seek the creative potential in our lives.

While studying or contemplating the ToL in KST we often aim to attain Keter, the highest state of consciousness. The irony is that once we achieve this high state of being there is nowhere to go but down even as we continue to go up. This descent can either go downward within the same ToL we have just climbed or it can go upward to the lowest part of the ToL above it.

(Refer back to the illustration, Five Elements of the Olamot Worlds.)

Beyond the Sephirah of Keter, we can connect with the Sephirah of Malchut of the ToL above. At that point Keter and Malchut become as one until they are not as one. Then, we enter Malchut with the seed of Keter below. Keter and Malchut are the same when they overlap and different when they do not overlap. This is mate-ve-lo-mate (truths that exist in contradiction) since they are the same yet different depending on their orientation in existence. That aspect of the ToL is mirrored in our DNA, whose repeated ladder like structure is the building block of life.

There are two primary ways of describing the supernal triad in relationship to each other. The first illustrates how the sephirot connect in time and space. Keter is viewed as a limitless point, Chochmah an infinite line and Binah a triangle. This matrix of creation is visualized as a geometric unfolding.

Within the body the view described above mirrors our individual experience in space time. When we connect with Keter, we are the center point within our perspective of the universe. Chochmah is the line that flows from the infinite point of Keter. This infinite line becomes many. These lines become arrows of time that radiate out in all directions around us as our past and future. Binah forms these arrows of time into an image that can be understood as our life. As we climb higher up the ToL our consciousness expands until we see our connection to other points, lines and forms until all becomes one.

The second way of describing the Supernal Triad's interpersonal expression is as mother and father. Keter is formless, Chochmah is a limitless point and Binah is a circle. The limitless point flows out toward

Binah, much the way a sperm swims toward an egg. The line enters the circle and fills it until it expands much the way the sperm connects with an egg. It is fertilized and the egg swells and differentiates into a form.

Both of the above descriptions attempt to convey a container, womb or vessel that helps birth our universe and transmit blessings. KST descriptions tend toward the first illustration since it is not bound to our reproductive abilities. Both views are correct. They are for our benefit of understanding that which is beyond our comprehension.

The sephirot of the supernal triad each have a secondary placement in the body. We study them further in the KSP level III classes.

BINAH

This delightfulness is the delight issuing from the world that is coming, and from the world that is going all lamps radiate, lights scattering everywhere. That goodness and radiance of the world that is coming, absorbed by the patriarchs, is called delightfulness.[19]

—*Zohar*, Daniel C. Matt

BINAH IS UNDERSTANDING IN HEBREW. Understanding is required for us to utilize the limitless wisdom that pours forth from Chochmah. Without understanding, there is no way to understand this process. Binah makes Chochmah's wisdom more accessible to us, similar to an editor clarifying a writer's thoughts for the reader.

In traditional Kabbalah, Binah is the third sephirah to become manifest. In KSTechnique, Binah is counted as the eighth sephirah since we are working with the physical body as the starting point toward healing.

Binah is the root-substance of form and the primordial formative influence. Through Binah are birthed the six sephirot, six directions, time, space and the four forces of nature. Binah also births the Sephirah of Malchut, the ultimate cause of the effect of creation. Binah plays a vital role in the cycle of life and death. She gives and takes life in the endless cycle of transformation. Binah is the primordial womb of the universe. It is the world of delight and connects us with our life's path in a dimension that exists beside us and inside of us, as truth.

Binah helps define our desires and intentions through thoughts and feelings, similar to how our brain contains thoughts. These thoughts enable us to make choices and visualize images. Binah is the understood part of wisdom. This understanding is found both in the brain's left hemisphere and secondarily in the heart.

The infinite points of Keter expand out in the lines of Chochmah, which are contained in the form of a triangle by Binah. The triangle of Binah is not physical but is the storehouse of energy from which we are nourished. Binah is the source of everything we want. Chochmah passively receives Keter's infinity; Binah actively shares it. All blessings come from the sharing of Binah.

Binah is King, reigning over all the lower Sephirot and also known as the Holy of Holies.[20]

—*Zohar*, Daniel C. Matt

Although Binah is often considered feminine, she contains a distinctly dual nature. Binah is sometimes called Elohim, which has a feminine beginning and a masculine/plural ending. This dualistic nature is also found in the blueprint of our genetics. Embryos have similar physical structures. We all begin as female. The existence of sex determining hormones will later trigger the development of male, female or a combination of genitalia.

Letters and Blessings

The Hebrew letters are symbols that facilitate the effects of the ohrim or healing energy in much the same way a prism refracts white light into a multi-colored rainbow. Each letter is assigned a number which makes up a system of numerology called gematria. The gematria value guides us with purpose and energy. The gematria for Binah is 50. Going through the 50 gates of the ToL is the path to Binah.

Traditional Hebrew prayers utilize the system of gametria to provide a key to understanding the blessings. First, we activate ZA, the central column on the ToL. Then we connect to Binah. We align our base desires with their spiritual counterparts in order to actively transform our desires into blessings.

Working with the energy of Binah can help bring blessings into our life. Use good judgment when receiving these blessings. Chaim Vital says that whoever seeks blessings is guaranteed to succeed regardless of our fate and circumstance. We just have to make the thresh hold of effort.

When we have a desire, we want to receive something. This is malchut consciousness. If we remain in that state of want the blessings that result will not be stable. We need to seek its opposite to stabilize our request. We balance our need to receive with our need to share. By restricting our desires through sharing, we bring the consciousness of Malchut's desires to Binah's so they can be sweetened and result in blessings. Our desires become stable. If our desire is left at the level of Malchut and is not sweetened, it may include judgment which results in uncomfortable situations.

In both situations our desires are met. With Binah's sweetness, blessings arrive in a form we ideally want. For instance, if we are tired and pray for a break to relax the blessing could come in the form of an illness that forces us to take a break. If our request is sweetened by Binah, we could end up with a Hawaiian vacation.

Receiving Binah's sweetened blessings through giving is mate-ve-lo-mate. By framing our desires to receive with giving we create a complete circuit of energy within our desires, sweetened and stable. By practicing restriction, we receive our desires in balance. We continue to climb the ToL, strive to earn the gematria value of 50 and reach for the blessings of Binah.

Details for Binah

Angel: none or seraphim
Animal: dove, raven
Archangel: none or Tzafkiel—sight of G-d, angel of understanding
Associated Earth element: oxygen
Body contact points: reflex zones / heart or middle of chest
Chief operating force: electromagnetism
Color: black or crimson
Dance movement: spring with arms up. Spin to the left. Stop and hold.
Yoga asana: rub hands together and place palms over eyes. Left palm to left hemisphere of head, right palm over heart
Direction: end
Element: fire
Essential oils: myrrh, tangerine, clary Sage
Finger: right thumb
Food: tomatoes, tomato juice, strawberry
Function: creation / destruction
Gematria: 50
Gems: onyx, smoky quartz
G-d's Name: YHVH (read Elohim)
Image: mature woman, vulva, chalice, veil, king
Inhabitant: throne of glory
Location: left hemisphere of the brain
Location on face: ears
Malfunction: loss of orientation in physical world
Matriarch: Leah
Meaning: understanding / great mother
Patriarch: none, as it is beyond human consciousness. Moses is the only patriarch to reach this level.
Planet: Saturn
Secondary placement: heart
Sense: hearing
Sound: Ay

Spelling of YHVH: YUD HY VAV HY (value 63)
Spiritual experience: sorrow of life which must be transcended
Tetragrammaton: upper Hey
Universe: Beriah (world of creation)
Vice: avarice
Virtue: silence
Vowel: Tzerey

Guided Visualization for Binah

Binah
Understanding
Black or Crimson
Fire
Thighs, Solar Plexus, Forehead
Obsidian

Allow darkness to envelope you. Let it cradle you. Nurture you. In this darkness you know yourself. Listen to your knowing. You know your purpose. But it seems just out of reach, just outside your conscious grasp. Your ears hear nothing. Your eyes are closed. You lie dreamless, not quite asleep, in the place where nothing and everything exists. Darkness is all around you now.

You float in clouds of emptiness, cradling you in peaceful darkness—nothing to hear, nothing to know. You are at peace. Feel the left side of your head. What does it feel like? What does it say? Gently allow the energy there to drift into your heart center. Breathe deeply into your heart, in the place between worlds, where your mind's heart speaks and hears. Listen to the sparkle of fiery light as it glistens through your darkness. It calls to you now. It is whispering your purpose. What does it say? Listen.

Breathe slowly. In and out... in and out... relax into yourself, relax into your body. Settle into its spaciousness, into the peaceful darkness inside. Become one with it. Become one within yourself. Let the darkness empty your mind as you become an infinity of form and light.

Rest in the womb of the void—the birthplace of your dreams to come.

A vibration caresses you in this darkness. A sound whispers in your inner ear, a movement, a flutter of a gentle wing across your breast, a warmth upon your heart, your ears, your head. It pulls. It rises and falls, then burns from nowhere. Be still. You are one. You are at peace.

A light glistens. A black and crimson rose opens. Watch it spin, open, embracing love and describing it, defining your purpose, a clarification for your pattern in this life. You call to the black-crimson light revealed.

Fear grips you. You are afraid to leave the womb of peaceful darkness, but the intuitive, black-crimson rose calls to your heart and mind. You are so hungry for answers. Your quest outward and inward, expanding, searching, learning, wanting more. You long to see more, to know, to surround yourself with the wonders around you. Its shapes, endless colors, multitude of forms. You heart and mind are filled with knowing recognition, the wonder of recognizing the safety and the peace the sound of light also brings.

Open your mind, open your heart, open your ears. See the black/crimson light brightening your way as you listen for its voice. What does it say? Observe the matter's solid form unwinding, seeking freedom on flames of truth. Open your mind. Your path now bright, heard by the heart. You have harnessed wisdom's thoughts to turn day to night and night to day.

The black - crimson rose spins. Other colors, shapes and forms reflect your purpose, answers your questions, shows you your life's patterns the way your mind and heart / heart and mind can clearly understand.

You mind opens. Your heart receives.

Contemplation Exercises for Binah

Following RT:
1. Contemplate the Hebrew letter Hey between your brows. Visualize it in black and crimson light drifting down to your heart center where it turns pink and green. Let it glow with

light, transform it without guidance. Then, consciously transform that light back to a black and crimson letter Hey between your brows.
2. Visualize yourself sitting in peaceful darkness while comfortable silence envelopes you. A ball of brilliant fire light approaches. Watch its waves oscillate, it's ripples venture forward and backward. These waves have a sound. What is that sound? Reach out and grab some of that fire light in your hands. It rests in your palms. Watch it glow, listen to its movements within your palms. Drink it into you—or let it go back into its endless waves of motion. Transform the waves into sound, as music. What did it feel like? What did it sound like? What did it say? How did it radiate within your body? How did it feel to let it go? Was there warmth? Burning? Cooling?
3. Sit in a steam room or sauna while performing RT for five to ten minutes.

CHOCHMAH

Paths of Wisdom[21]

—*Sefer Yetzirah*, Aryan Kaplan

CHOCHMAH IS WISDOM IN HEBREW. We connect with and appreciate our ineffable, nonverbal nature in the Sephirah of Chochmah. Kabbalah repeatedly states that the sephirot must be reached by paths of wisdom. Follow these paths to access these greater and greater spiritual heights: the paths of nonverbal chochmah consciousness.

Binah is the divine mother, Chochmah the divine father and Keter the crown that rests upon them. Chochmah connects to our physical eyes. It facilitates true sharing and is a primary channel for the light of the ohrim. When we are joined at this level, we exist in unity with love and light. We only desire to share and be one with the universe. In chochmah consciousness, we lose free will.

However, if we have climbed the thirty-two paths of wisdom found in the ToL (Tree of Life), then we will have learned their lessons. We maintain our sense of individuality within the bliss of the limitless light of the ohrim as found in Chochmah.

The number thirty-two is represented by the culmination of the twenty-two symbols that are the consonants found in the Hebrew alphabet along with the ten dimensions found as Hebrew's ten vowels. These represent the thirty-two paths that are all about channeling energy.

The energy of Chochmah flows constantly. If Keter is a point, Chochmah becomes a line, or the extension of an infinite point. There are infinite lines that flow forth from each infinite point. Within these lines reside complete and infinite wisdom.

Chochmah is like a superconductor for electricity. The best superconductor known on earth is gold, but it is too expensive to use as electrical wiring. If Chochmah was gold, the other sephirot would be the other metals and would provide different rates and qualities of flow. Each flow has a place and quality it can share that goes beyond its capacity for channeling energy. We work with the sephirot that match our own frequency. The sephirot meet us and help us journey on our life's path toward Chochmah's wisdom and ultimate *bittul* (humility).

When we achieve humility, we transcend to spiritual heights without losing our sense of individuality. Humility offers us a stable vessel to contain the energy. To be exposed to the large flow of current found in Chochmah before we are ready would mean burning up without purpose. We need a stable vessel.

Limitless wisdom flows through the Sephirah of Chochmah. When we are completely open within a stable vessel, devoid of ego and have no desires, we are ready to receive Chochmah. We cannot sustain the consciousness of Chochmah while in human form as it is beyond our ability. We can seek to understand and connect to this wisdom through practice. No human being can completely reach this level since we will always have wants, even if that want only extends to the air we breathe. Give up the desire for air and we will no longer exist in human form.

It is not our purpose to stay in chochmah consciousness indefinitely. We are meant to have a human experience. Seek to connect with the

Sephirah of Chochmah. Understand and integrate its wisdom into our lives. This is how we can catch a glimpse of Chochmah.

We are the most accepting of Chochmah energy when we feel crushed by life's struggles. When our ego attachment falls away, we are humble. We do not need to destroy our lives on purpose. Through conscious practice, contemplation and meditation we have the opportunity to detach from ego and experience Chochmah. There are various KST, Kabbalistic, Native American and Ayurvedic techniques that can facilitate this practice.

Even with these techniques, bad things may happen. At that point, we can make Chochmah part of our spiritual journey.

In KST, Chochmah is counted as the ninth sephirot. But in traditional Kabbalah, Chochmah is the second sephirah since it was the second of the sephirot to become manifest in creation.

Chochmah gives of its wisdom with no reservation or thought. It expands with boundless desire as it begins dispersing the limitless energy of Keter. This energy provides divine stimulation for the arts, for love and for creation unbound. We elevate sparks and connect with this energy when participating in our life's talents.

A vessel is a term that describes the forms within creation that are able to contain spiritual light. Vessel consciousness refers to our ability to contain spiritual light. The beginning of vessel consciousness begins at Chochmah, where creation begins to have form. This energy is associated with the highest of the four levels of creation, known as Atzilut, where time and space break down. Past, present and future are accessible here. When our ego has been crushed or its voice quieted, we can connect to this energy more easily. We receive guidance. Our lives may not shift immediately. But if we integrate this energy into our lives, we will keep its wisdom even as our ego consciousness returns.

Part of human nature is searching for the easiest path. For instance, while working at ashrams or other spiritual centers we often have chores that we dislike. It seems that if we don't like washing sheets, we are given the opportunity to connect with Chochmah by being in a situation where we have to wash sheets. We continue to wash until we have surrendered to the flow of Chochmah. We truly connect when we no longer hate the chore. We are released from the suffering. Then we may be given another opportunity to connect with the energy of Chochmah.

When the energy of Chochmah is flowing into our life and is met with resistance we become blocked. When Henry David Thoreau said that, "The mass of men lead lives of quiet desperation and go to the grave with the song still in them,"[22] it was as though he was referring to that state of ego where Chochmah cannot flow.

If there is fear associated with how Chochmah is manifesting in life, try and allow space for the fear to move. Fear is often the culprit of our not wanting to receive Chochmah. Reframing our fear helps. The word for awe in the Tanakh is often translated as fear. Awe may contain an element of fear but it is combined with love. We may begin with fear. But if we fear learning, fear walking the first steps, we will never move forward. Perhaps we fear not getting the results we want. For instance, we study the names of the ten sephirot for fear of not passing a KST test. But eventually, we walk in a path of love. In the case of the test, after memorizing the names and attributes of the sephirot, we will love them and want to delve further!

We experience fear when we are uncertain; uncertain about our environment and about our safety. Fear without a trigger can be about the uncertainty of the physical body that takes the form of survival of our vessel. Transcending these fears infuses our lives with light and love. We develop stability and a connection to our true nature and purpose.

Details for Chochmah

Angel: none or Akatriel—angel of the presence
Animal: hawk
Associated Earth element: uranium
Inhabitant: sephirot

Archangel: none or Ratziel—guider of the creative force or soul
Body contact points: reflex zones
Chief operating force: strong nuclear force. Pionic force.
Color: grey or pure soft blue
Dance movements: flowing grapevine. Spin to right, stop and hold
Yoga asana: palm over parietals. right palm to right hemisphere of head, left palm over heart
Direction: beginning
Element: Water
Essential oils: musk, frankincense, vetiver, blue tansy, lavender
Finger: right index finger
Food: apple, pear, (sweet fruits), tisane teas
Function: expansion
Gems: labradorite, aquamarine
G-d's name: Yah / The Eternal
Image: father, thunderbolt, line
Location: right hemisphere of brain
Location on face: eyes
Malfunction: ignorance
Meaning: wisdom
Patriarch: none
Planet: Uranus
Second placement: point below navel
Sense: sight
Sound: Ah
Spelling of YHVH: YUD HY VYV HY (value = 72)
Spiritual experience: unification experience. Vision of G-d
Tetragrammaton: Yud
Universe: Atzilut (realm of pure divinity)
Vice: no-vice
Virtue: devotion
Vowel: Patach

Guided Visualization for Chochmah

Chochmah Wisdom
Grey
Water
Feet, Pelvis, Chest,
Labradorite
Expansiveness, Intellect and Linear Thinking

Rest now.

Let your breath flow in... and out... in... and out...

Be a droplet in your deep moving sea. Infinity. A radiance of mind complete.

Relax into yourself, relax into the right side of your head. What does the energy there feel like? Allow that energy to connect with the space between your eyebrows. Allow yourself to gently settle into that point and wade through the space between your brows.

Watch that infinite point as it expands into an infinite line, connecting with the point just a hairbreadth below your belly button. Another point reaches back to your brown and the circuit of light begins to flow, reaching for the stars, reaching out in every direction... expanding into flowing spaciousness. It pulls. It rises and falls, then flows from nowhere. Be a droplet in your deep moving sea. Infinity. A flow of mind complete. Be still. You are one. You are at peace.

The water glistens. A translucent blue-gray line calls to you from the center of your brow. Watch it flow outward in all directions, open, as the water-filled grey rose ascends, opens, swirls... showing you direction, guidance, the wisdom of your higher self whispers its wisdom, wanting you to hear.

Expand your thoughts, ever weaving wisdom's webs with timeless patterns. You flow and ebb... in bliss.

The rose calls for your intellect to awaken, your intelligence to know truth, a call to memory, the call of the translucent blue-gray rose revealed. Open your mind. Open your eyes. See the blue-gray dewy rose illuminate your path. What do you see?

These endless points of wisdom guide you—inward, outward. They surround you—endlessly interweaving, dancing, flowing in divine rhythm. The gray rose spins, showing you direction, guidance. The wisdom of your higher self whispers, wanting you to hear.

Other blue-gray roses flow, reflecting your purpose, answering questions in their river of never-ending wisdom, showing you your life's way that your mind can grasp. Your mind opens. Your bodies intuition opens. Your mind receives.

But the gray rose flows endlessly. Its color expands, changes, brightens, ebbs and flows. There is too much flow. Overwhelming. Cascading. Drowning. You call for help.

Immediately it softens. Wisdoms flow softens. The rushing river becomes a gentle stream, caressing, cradling the softness of the blue-gray rose petal caressing your temples. Your inner vision reaches out, seeing truth, removing doubt. See yourself open inside and watch, as the blue-gray rose spins again. Watch as your wisdom's flow guides your path. Our life's purpose is revealed.

Within your brow, within the blue-grey, you know your way.

Contemplation Exercises for Chochmah

Following RT:
1. Sit comfortably and quietly. Close your eyes. Visualize the letter Yud between your brows. Let it flow with expansive fluid light, transform at will into whatever it wants. Then, consciously bring that light back to a Yud between your brows.

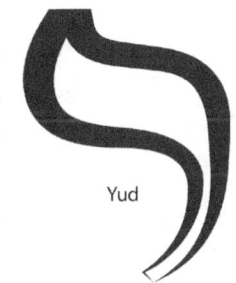
Yud

2. Visualize an infinite point in space. See this point slowly expand out into a line. The line extends out to infinity. See another line extending out from the original point,

and another and another, radiating in all directions—limitless. How does this feel to you? What message can be found in this limitless linear extension? Another point appears. A limitless line draws forth from this point as well, followed by another, and another. How can these lines all be extending out from multiple points that are, each of them, the center of our universe? Be open to the answers.
3. Perform RT during a shirodharah treatment, while water cascades of your head or with cool mist from a humidifier drifting over your head.
4. When you eat, become conscious of each bite. Contemplate your thirty-two teeth as the thirty-two paths of Chochmah. Separate the negativity from the positivity of your food. How does the food taste and feel in your mouth? Be aware. Imagine the light that elevates you as you begin to digest this food.
5. Next time you find yourself in a situation you do not like, tell yourself you love it! How does your reaction change?
6. Number 5 can also be performed in the form of a contemplative meditation. Close your eyes and imagine doing something positive that you do not like to do. Visualize it in your mind. Now shift your consciousness to that of love. You love it! Do it with love.

KETER

The highest faculty in man is will.[23]

—Sefer Yetzirah, Aryan Kaplan

KETER MEANS CROWN IN HEBREW. As the crown, Keter is at the very top of the ToL. This is significant since Malchut represents kingdom. The crown determines the kingdom just as the kingdom is the purpose of the crown.

It was the first sephirah to manifest in creation. All other sephirotic potentials are contained within Keter. This subtlest of the sephirot provides the backdrop for all life experiences. Keter transcends all the laws of manifestation that result from this creation. Our human form is unable to fully grasp this level.

Keter is the observer. This sephirah is the reflection of Ein Sof or the unmanifest infinite. Keter's energy is analogous to pure being, without division. We can imagine Keter as a point in the center of the universe. There are an infinite number of these points. The point has no mass, depth or dimension, yet, this point is limitless, transcending time and space as we know it. Keter is hidden intelligence. It is found in everything yet remains invisible to us. Keter is pure being without activity.

The closest we can come to understanding Keter is mate-ve-lo-mate. It both exists but doesn't exist. If we can understand Keter then we don't "get it," nevertheless, we should try to understand.

Each ToL connects with another. When connecting to a subsequent ToL, the Sephirah of Keter of the first tree becomes the Sephirah of Malchut of the one above it. Likewise, the Malchut of the first tree connects to the Keter of the one below it. Although represented as a separate ToL in diagrams, they are actually reflections of one another. All of the sephirot are reflected in Malchut whereas all of the sephirot are contained in Keter while reflecting Ein Sof. The bridge between these two sephirot are the connection points within all of creation. *(Refer back to illustration: Five Levels of the Olamot Worlds.)*

Within our human consciousness we have choice. When we experience something in our lives, we can either choose to see it through keter consciousness or malchut consciousness. Putting the lower case name of the sephirah before the term consciousness defines our state of consciousness. Keter and malchut consciousness can both exist simultaneously but we are only capable of experiencing one at a time.

Malchut, the consciousness of emptiness, reflects judgment based on the physical universe. Alternatively, keter consciousness will feel full, bright and expansive. We can choose either to focus on emptiness and loss or the optimism that exists by being a component of the ToL.

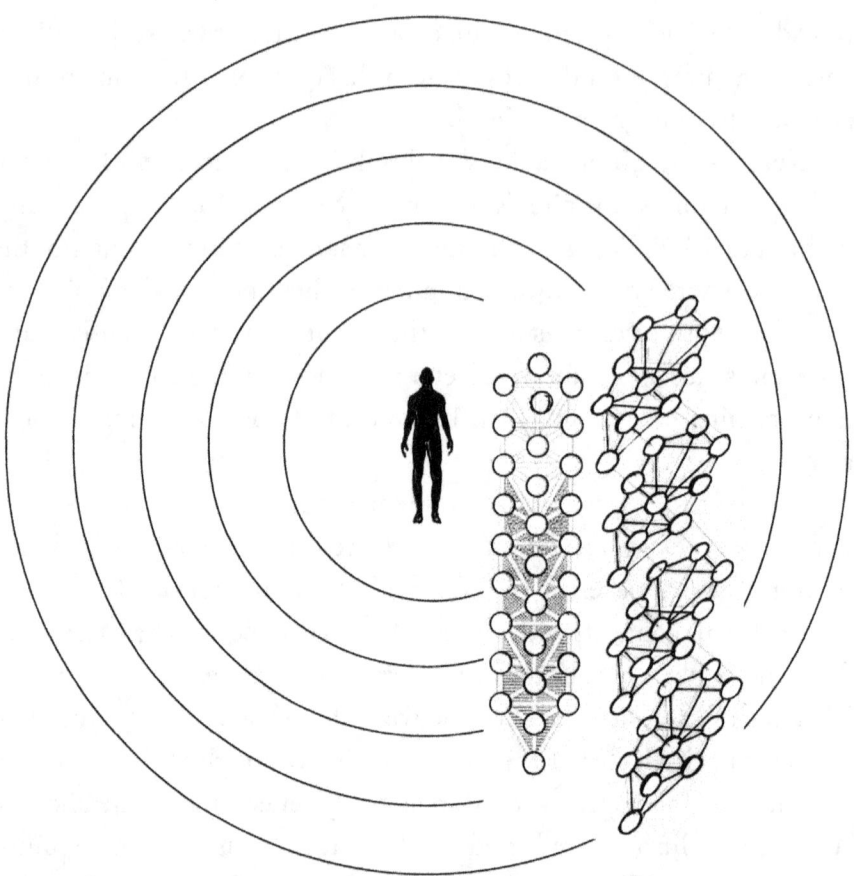

More specifically, we can either choose to be empty with the loss of something or we can be optimistic that space is needed to make room for something good.

Keter and malchut consciousness exist within each experience. We embrace both, feel them and allow movement between them. This processing is imperative in order to arrive at keter consciousness. In choosing keter consciousness without denying Malchut's reflection, we create a balance. To understand that both Keter and Malchut are reflections of each other yet opposites is mate-ve-lo-mate, knowing and not knowing simultaneously.

There are two types of spiritual light described in traditional Kabbalah. They are the inner light and the surrounding light, called makif and panimi. The inner light is the wisdom that we have inside of us. It is the light of the upper worlds reflecting upon the lower physical World of Asiyah. The surrounding light is the light that envelopes us and partners with us. We become receptive to the light's comfort. Both forms of light are part of the ohrim, the universal healing light.

Surrounding light can cause us to feel pressure to achieve. This is Keter signaling us to change for our higher good. The force impacts all the other sephirot. We feel unsatisfied, yearning to have more. Keter doesn't let us be comfortable in the bliss of the light for long. Our search for comfort only leads to chaos. Complacency will not allow achievement. Keter pushes us towards perfection because the light of Keter wants to give us everything.

Constraining the energy of Keter—the surrounding light—requires balance. We restrict our desire. Instead of acting impulsively, we wait for the rush of desire to subside. By practicing restriction we are actively working in relationship with creation. We receive our desire without a short circuit. Life becomes easier, less dramatic. Restricting our desires is living in unison with Keter and Malchut.

Details for Keter

Angel: None or Hyos Ha Kodoish—the highest servant
Animal: swan, eagle
Archangel: None or Metatron (scribe angel)
Associated Earth element: metal, hydrogen
Body contact points: reflex zones
Chief operating force: weak Nuclear Force
Color: white/ brilliance / absence of color when hidden
Dance movements: unwinding beginning standing up with arms and hands above or on the top of the head
Direction: none
Element: aether
Essential oils: rose, sandalwood, white lotus
Finger: right thumb

Food: none
Function: to facilitate our life's purpose
Gems: diamond, clear quartz
G-d's Name: Ehyeh Asher Ehyeh / I Am That I Am
Image: lamp, point, crown, ouroboros
Level or world: Yechida / Adam Kadmon
Location: crown of head / skull
Location on face: none / overall
Malfunction: feeling of disconnection from life and life's purpose
Meaning: crown
Patriarch: none
Planet: Pluto
Secondary placement: third eye between the brows
Sense: will
Sound: Ah, Aw
Spelling of YHVH: all
Spiritual Experience: union with and knowledge of the All
Tetragrammaton: tip of yud
Vice: none
Virtue: attainment and completion of an individual's life purpose.
Vowel: Kametz
Yoga asana: dead body pose

Guided Visualization for Keter

Crown
White
Aether
Reflex Points
Clear Quartz
Consciousness, Connection with your Higher Self

The white rose opens. Feel yourself expand into its light, into your light as the white rose opens.

Your journey... it is complete and has just begun. You have tasted, you have moved with the rhythm of your own self remembered. You have seen, you have felt into your own vibration, the light is the key that has opened your conscious eye...

And now you open into yourself, your higher self, supported by petals of light, the petals of the ohrim beneath you, around you, becoming one with you.

Feel the love you have felt, the loss of it, the returning of it.

Love.

Open to its meaning, let it guide you to your purpose.

Divine love opens. Supported by a thousand rose petals.

You have arrived back to your beginnings. Home. One.

Your journey is almost complete. There is but one small step... so small yet it will take you the farthest. That smallest step... take it... trust it... yes divine one, it is such a small step, because you are already there... you have always been there.

Be ready and open this last rose, one more light. Open it now. See the white light of the ohrim spin and open. Watch and let the light combine and be your small step to all that lies within you.

Feel the light bathe you. Try not to contain it. Just be. Be in the mystery of your own self remembered.

Rest now. Rest in the memory of your own journey. Remember the solidity of the earth, the flow of water through your body, the fire of power in your belly, the wind of love in your heart, the vibration in your throat, the visions in your mind's sight.

Remember now. Remember your journey into your body, into your self, into your life and beyond.

How do you feel about having been on this journey? What has helped you on your journey? Your guidance is present for you.

All wisdom is within you. Nothing is beyond your awareness. Feel all that is before you, within you and around you. All wisdom is your mind, is your body, is your spirit, is your essence. You are but a drop in a sea of bliss, connected with so many, related, divine, intelligence revealed.

Let the patterns of creation, your own divine creation, with its vastness, with its infinity, surround you. Let it envelope you in white, opalescent mist nourish you. Feel the white rose that blooms atop your head. Opening. Sense it. Know it. Feel illuminated by it. Let it connect you with heaven and earth.

Find the white rose flower in you.

You exist beyond form—above it, around it, behind it, within it, without and through it all you ARE.

You have come full circle on your journey and the pattern you have created is complete.

Watch, as the white, opalescent rose spins with white radiating from its petaled tips. Magnificent. Deep within the rose you find the sacred space to open your mind. Open it now. Reach towards the flower. Reach out beyond the veil of illusion. Fly over the starlit trail before you now.

Your primal knowing within speaks now. Listen from your sacred place where you began and where, ending, you shall return. Reconnect to your bliss and trust yourself.

Open to the divinity within you now. The white rose is open. Know it, and you will bring it forth with peaceful presence, a knowing purpose, the white rose, ever present, ever loving.

Your white rose is your gateway to the worlds within, without and the worlds beyond. In this sacred space and gentle peace, you open. Connected. It is all one. Love. Wisdom. Peace.

Let the sacred rose light your way.

Contemplation Exercises for Keter

Following RT:

1. Sit, quietly contemplating a contradiction and/or paradox of life. What does the term mate-ve-lo mate mean in your life? Some examples:
    a. Anti-matter within our universe of matter.
    b. Divine love in the world where pain exists.
    c. Unrequited desire within a world of limitless potential.

2. Visualize a point in space. See this point as the center of the universe. Another point appears which is also the center of our known universe. Continue to add these paradoxical points to your visualization. Experience each of them as limitless, ever expanding, ever present and in every aspect of this creation. Ask yourself this question: How can the center of all things exist everywhere all at once?
3. Breathe and meditate with any question you may have. Open yourself. Be a channel. Be a conduit for healing. Then, write a question. Be completely open to the answer that is meant for you. Be open to the answer.

Chapter 8

Sephirot Revisted

Ten Sephirot of nothingness, ten and not nine, ten and not eleven. [24]
—*Sefer Yetzirah,* Ayreh Kaplan

We were introduced to the details of the sephirot in chapter three. Now, we review and learn how to see the ToL in all things including within our own body and in others. In doing so we begin to listen to what our body is telling us on a subtle level. Self-knowledge enables us to be a clear channel for others. For instance, increasing awareness of our unconscious nature as found in the Sephirah of Netzach helps us to differentiate ourselves from another. This makes it easier to walk in another's shoes without losing our sense of self. In turn, we generate the greater level of empathy that is found in the Sephirah of Hod.

The sephirot are the building blocks of creation. The pathways between and among them represent the different ways the sephirot connect and interact. How we interact with the sephirot shows us our personal progression on the ToL. Being able to identify where we are on the ToL helps us be more aware of where we are in our life so that we can make conscious choices about our life. We can see where we are going and compare it to our ideal of where we would like to go.

From the highest perspective there is no separation. The sephirot are interconnected. To study different parts of the whole by making distinctions between the sephirot is for our own sake. It is meant to help us traverse the entirety of creation in a way that we can understand. For instance, in Kabbalah the sephirot are traditionally described from top down starting with the Sephirah of Keter and ending with the Sephirah of Malchut. In KSTechnique® we begin most readings of the sephirot of the ToL (Tree of Life) from bottom up rather than up to bottom. We read the sephirot in the body from Malchut to Keter. This is because we are beginning from where we are at this moment. We are physical beings reaching up toward higher and more expansive states of consciousness. We are going from the effect of creation to the origin of creation or from our body, as matter, to the beginnings of it, as energy.

From the perspective of Ein Sof (infinite) there is no distinction between the Sephirot of Keter and Malchut, between energy and matter, between the spiritual and the mundane. Ein Sof is mirrored in oneness whereby above and below are the same. However, Ein Sof is both oneness itself and beyond oneness. To know this state is beyond human capability. Mate-ve-lo-mate is as close as we can come to understanding Ein Sof. Our feeling of separation from Ein Sof is what gives us freedom of choice and allows us to grow and mature as individuals. As we grow, we become conscious, able to exist in the bliss of knowing the whole, while still maintaining a sense of individuality.

SEPHIROT IN THE BODY

THE SEPHIROT ACT AS A BRIDGE for the universal healing light of the ohrim. Rarely does anything in the universe take place except through the medium of the sephirot. The sephirot are understood as an expression of Ein Sof but not Ein Sof. From the perspective of Ein Sof, even the sephirot are beli-mah, meaning "nothingness," or literally "without anything," even though they make up everything.

Getting to know the sephirot in the body starts with learning about the esoteric anatomy and physiology. Esoteric anatomy refers to the structure of our energy field. Esoteric physiology refers to how the energy field interfaces with itself, the physical body and the environment. Studying these systems is similar to the study of standard anatomy and physiology.

The sephirot of the ToL found in the body are a part of our esoteric anatomy. Studying the sephirot as energy centers within our bodies will help us learn the language and purpose of them in our lives.

Sephirot are the basic mode of creative power in the body. Once we know which sephirah correlate to which part of the body we can gain insight into what their frequency is telling us. This does not mean that the sephirot are those parts of the body. Rather the energy of certain parts of our body vibrate at a frequency that is compatible with the frequency of a certain sephirah. We can access their energy more readily from these designated locations. The frequency of the body part is a key to unlock the door of a particular sephirah.

Since most of the sephiric energy is not measurable by today's means, it is easier to imagine their energy in a way we can relate to. Kabbalah calls this type of anthropomorphizing of the sephirot within the body a partzuf. We make an undefinable part of creation definable by making it accessible to our consciousness.

By anthropomorphizing the energy of the sephirot we better focus our kavana (intention) to facilitate healing within the body. The partzuf for the Supernal Triad of Keter, Chochmah and Binah is called Arich Anpin (long face). The partzuf of the six emotional Sephirot of Chesed through Yesod is called ZA (Zeir Anpin or small face).

From our perspective the ToL and esoteric anatomy may appear different among cultures but from a wider perspective they are all similar. It may go by different names and partzufim but it is still the ToL. For instance, Yesod's placement on the ToL is the Hara in Ayurveda and Dan Tien in Chinese Medicine. The three pillars of the ToL is the caduceus of western medicine and the Ida, Pingala and Sushumna Nadi's of Ayurveda.

Sephirotic Body Map

Following are maps of the ToL within the body. They are used by KST practitioners when reading the sephirot of the ToL in the body.

KSTechnique® I map for reading the front of the body:

> Malchut is found at the feet
> Yesod is found between the navel and pubis
> Hod is found at the left knee
> Netzach is found at the right knee
> Tipheret is found at the solar plexus
> Gevurah is found at the left arm (shoulder to palm)
> Chesed is found at the right arm (shoulder to palm)
> Binah is found at the left side of the head
> Chochmah is found at the right side of the head
> Keter is found just above the center of the head

KSTechnique® I map for reading the back of the body:

> KSTechnique® I reading map of the back of the body:
> Malchut is found at the coccyx
> Yesod is found at the crux of the back
> Hod is found at the left kidney
> Netzach is found at the right kidney
> Tipheret is found at the mid back
> Gevurah is found at the left arm (shoulder to palm)
> Chesed is found at the right arm (shoulder to palm)
> Binah is found at the left side of the head
> Chochmah is found at the right side of the head
> Keter is found above the center of the head

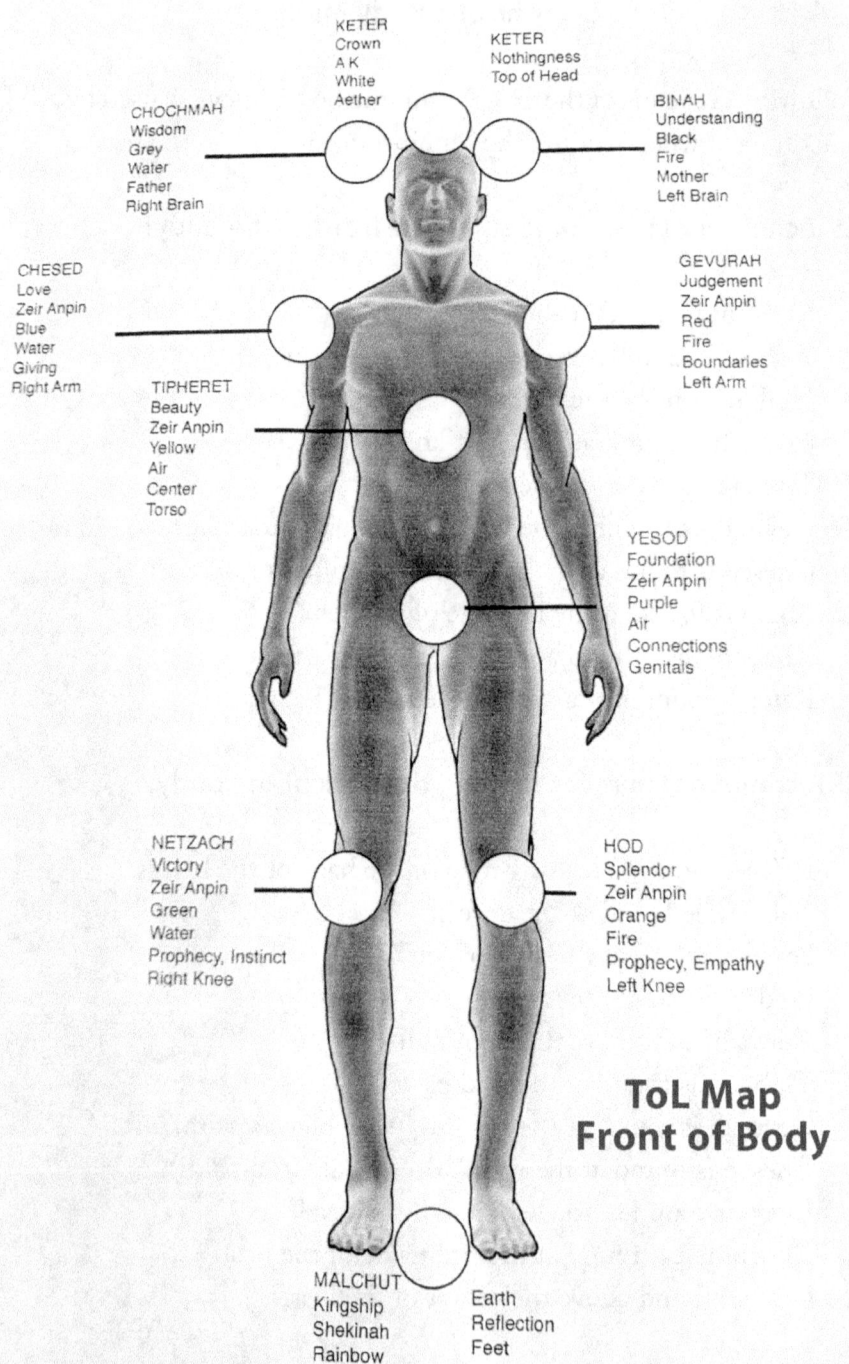

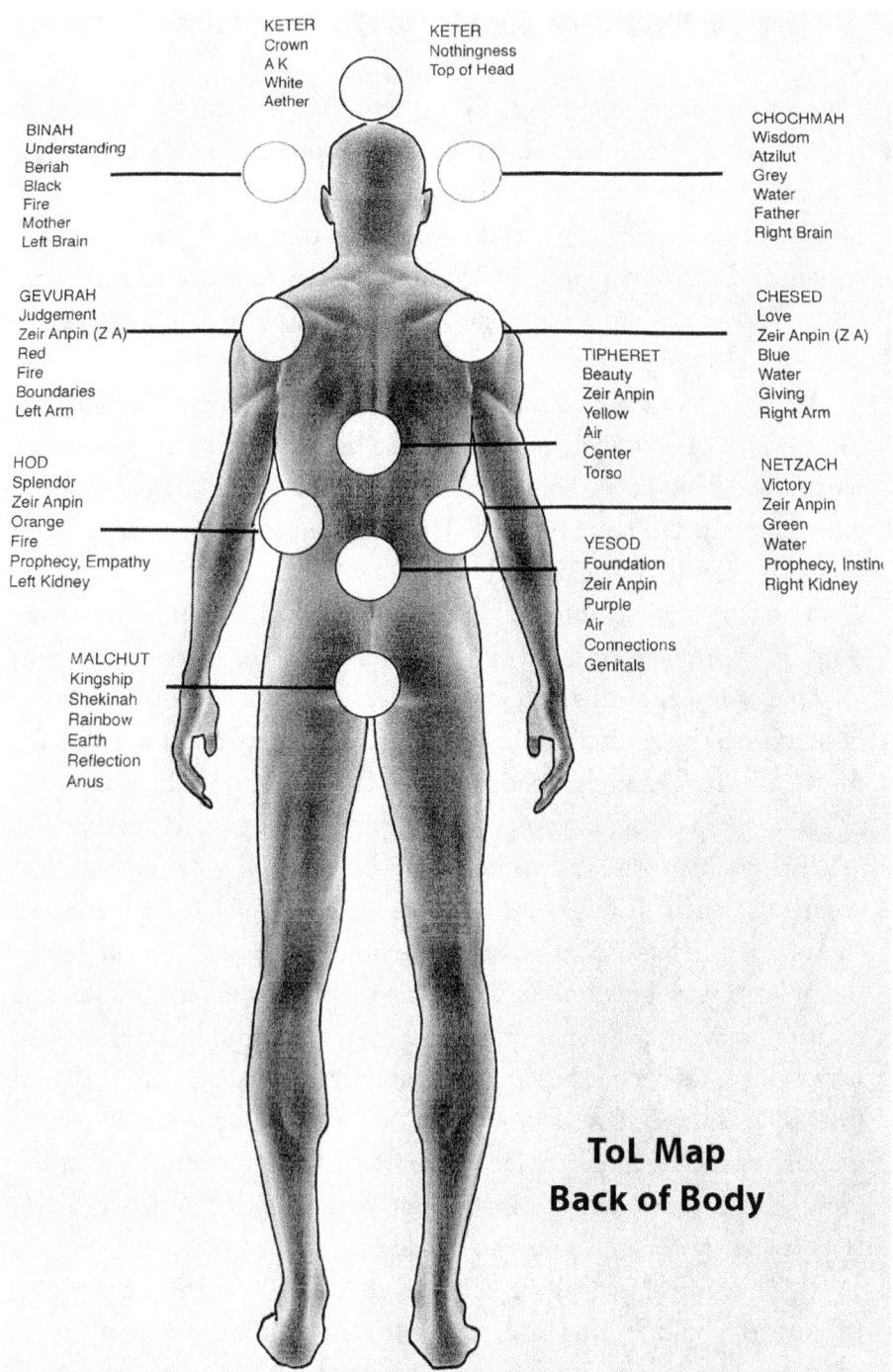

ToL Map Back of Body

Why are Sephirotic Readings for the Front and Back Different?

The configuration of the ToL for the front and back of the body shift in order to accommodate our structure. This protects us while allowing for optimal mobility and personal growth. The overwhelming power of infinity has far more energy and information than our human form can sustain and still remain human. We are simply not created to withstand that amount of energy without getting seriously burned. It is not a good or a bad thing. It simply is.

When we are looking forward we are facing the light. The light of the sephirot can overwhelm us. This also holds true for the light of the ohrim. The front of the body is far more cognizant of light and shadow. Therefore, the structure of the ToL is augmented more in the front of the body than the back of the body.

The ohrim is the universal healing light of Infinity. It is an unconditional expression of a desire to heal. As practitioners we want to channel as much of this light as is needed during a session. When we hold space by being present during a KST session we become a channel for the ohrim. Through practice we can handle more and more of this light. We prepare our body without burning ourselves out of existence.

Imagine two paintings. The first is called, "Enlightenment." The second is called, "Enlightenment Before Its Time." Enlightenment shows a person floating, rainbow colors vibrating through, arms stretching upward with joy on their face. This is the blissful effect of being a prepared vessel for the energy of the ohrim. The second painting is of a person who has been exposed to the same energy but was not prepared for it. The same rainbow colors course through their body but their arms are mangled at their torso, face is contorted and feet crushed on the ground. The same energy flows through both images. How we respond to that energy depends upon how ready we are to receive it.

It is like infusing a 40-watt light bulb with 120 watts of electricity. It burns the bulb. In this case, we are the bulb. In order to prepare for more healing energy, we practice techniques that will strengthen our vessels, body and mind.

The mystic, endowed with native talents for this sort of thing and following, stage by stage, the instruction of a master, enters the waters and finds he can swim; whereas the schizophrenic, unprepared, unguided, and ungifted, has fallen or has intentionally plunged, and is drowning. [25]
— Myths to Live By, Joseph Campbell

Joseph Campbell's observation is one of the mysteries touched on in ancient Kabbalist texts. The synopsis that is repeated throughout these manuscripts is that to come face to face with infinity directly is to be obliterated. In the Tanakh it is only Moses who was able to face G-d directly and he never was the same afterwards. However, even Moses faced G-d at the level of Elohim, which is the level of G-d within nature. There were higher frequencies of G-d's name yet to meet.

THE PENDULUM

USING HEALING TOOLS IS A GOOD WAY to access different methods of healing without overwhelming our own esoteric anatomy. The pendulum is one of the easiest healing tools for learning how to read energy. In KST protocols, the pendulum is a tool to read the sephirot as energy centers in the body.

It is composed of an evenly weighted item called a pendant that is attached to a flexible chain or string. The item can be anything from a crystal to a paper clip. Crystals as pendants can be both healing and aesthetically appealing but they are not necessary. It is up to us as practitioners to decide what works best for us.

The chain of the pendulum needs to be long enough to comfortably wrap around our finger a few times and still allow for at least 6 to 8 inches between our finger and the pendant. The chain needs to be flexible and attached to the center of the weighted item so that the pendant can move freely.

How the Pendulum Works

Working with the pendulum can feel mysterious. It seems to move on its own during a reading. Once we understand how the pendulum works the mystery dissolves. Get comfortable with the mechanics of the pendulum in order to keep things as simple as possible. This will help give an objective reading. When doing a KST protocol with a pendulum a circuit of communication is established.

We start with learning how to hold the pendulum. Wrap the end of the pendulums chain around the distal part of the middle finger three times. We hold our hand over the area we want to read. The weighted item should be three to six inches above the body if we are assessing the Body of Yezirah or the emotional body. This is the most common part of the esoteric anatomy to read during a session. A detailed description of the layers of the esoteric anatomy are covered more fully in the chapter eleven.

Once the reading starts, hold space and remember the client's kavana or intention for the session. A client's kavana is assessed during the intake part of a KST session. The pendulum will begin to move. This is a result of the client's energy flow in the area being read. Observe the movement of the pendulum and how it relates to the area you are reading.

Tell the client your assessment. Ask the client if the reading resonates with them. As the reading progresses, more energy begins to move. This can be experienced by the client as awareness, shaking, crying, remaining quiet, giggling, talking, chattering, falling asleep or any manner of change. Work on that area if indicated or continue to the next energy center to be read.

Usually the treatment portion of the session does not officially begin until after the entire ToL reading but there are exceptions. A complete circuit of communication is made once the pendulums movement is explained to the client and the client processes and responds to the information.

Our body has extremely intricate senses. They continuously input information on both a gross and energetic level. This sensory information is passed onto our subconscious where it is processed on an instinctual level. A lesser amount of this information goes to our conscious mind. Using the pendulum during a reading is one way to gain access to the information stored in the subconscious.

During a session a client may ask if the practitioner is moving the pendulum themselves. The answer is yes and no. The delicate, unconscious reactions within the body's musculature and energy field generate the pendulum's oscillations. Although unconscious, the movements are made by us. These movements create an avenue for transmitting subtle information to our conscious mind, which we may then knowingly work with and verbalize to our client.

Working with the pendulum is an amazing experience. We become aware of your body's ability to receive and transmit information that lies beyond our conscious awareness. Around eighty-five percent of our actions are driven by our subconscious or unconscious. Yet, our body/mind/spirit has the ability to encompass it all. The pendulum is one of the many tools to help us access a bit of the information that lies beyond our awareness.

The Pendulum and the Heart

We want to remain open to our client during a KST session. Hold the pendulum in the hand that will allow our body mechanics to be open to the client's energy. Position the heart center so that it is open to our client's heart center. For instance, if we are on our client's right side, we will want to hold the pendulum with our right hand while reading Malchut (sephirah one at the feet) through Chesed (sephirah seven at right arm) or Da'at (sephirah at occiput). Change hands and hold the pendulum with the left hand while reading Binah (sephirah eight at the head) through Keter (sephirah ten at the top of head). If we move to the opposite side of the body during the reading of the Supernal Triad we do not need to change the pendulum to the other hand.

Language of the Pendulum

Once we connect with a sephirah during a KST reading the pendulum will begin to move in a way that describes the general state of that sephirah in the client's body. The pendulum will make different patterns during a ToL reading. Each pattern represents a different state of the sephirah being read. It is the language of the pendulum. We learn this language in order to better communicate with our client. The meanings of the different movements are listed below:

Clockwise: Open and flowing in a good direction. This is a balanced, healthy and positive pattern.
Counter Clockwise: Energy is flowing in a negative direction. Energy is being redirected from its intended course. The client may want to asses what issues may be causing the negative flow.
No Movement: Energy is blocked or stuck.
Vibration: Energy is trying to flow but there is an obstruction preventing it. The energy is sputtering out like a garden hose that has a block or kink in it. When the water is turned on, the hose will spray the water and pressure is felt at the block. In this case, the obstruction is in the esoteric anatomy of the client.
Vertical (up and down from head to feet): Cut off in communication between masculine and feminine, the rational and abstract and the active and receptive respectively.
Horizontal (from left to right): Cut off between heaven and earth, between the higher and lower sephirot. This represents a disconnect between what the client wants their life to look like (in relation to the meaning of the sephirah being read) and what the client's life looks like in the physical world.
Diagonal (from right shoulder to left hip): Logistical or rational issue.
Diagonal (from left shoulder to right hip): Emotional issue.
Continues to change directions: Confusion.
Two directions: The meaning of both directions are influencing the sephirah being read.

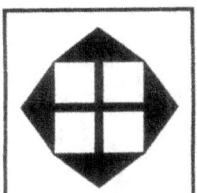
Two Directions
Both directions
are issues

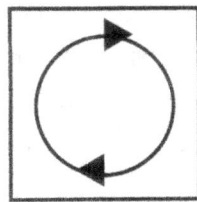
Clockwise
Balance

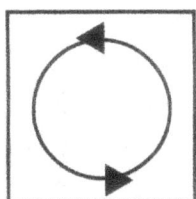
Counter
Clockwise
Negative flow

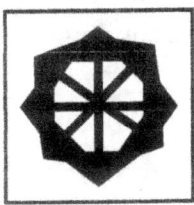
Changes Direction
Confusion

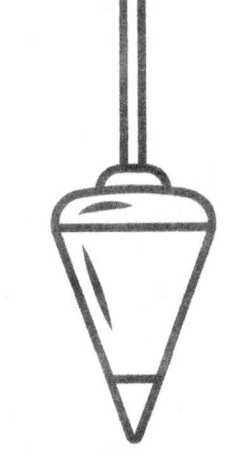

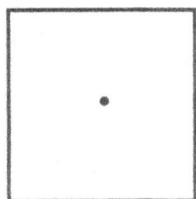
No Movement
Blocked

Left Diagonal
Emotional issue

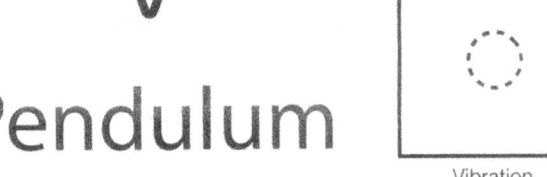
Vibration
Obstruction

Right Diagonal
Rational issue

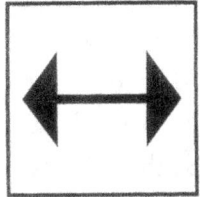
Horizontal
Cute off between
heaven and earth

Vertical
Cut off between
rational and abstract

SCANNING

DURING SCANNING WE USE OUR HANDS to detect energy flow. This is the second way KST practitioners learn to read the sephirot in the body. This technique works like the pendulum to assess a client's energy field... without the pendulum.

We begin by holding space and infusing our palms with ohrim. Place open palms over the area to be read. Allow the energy of the ohrim to guide you. In the second and third KSP classes the healing energy can be further enhanced through an attunement. Other techniques include drawing healing symbols or connecting with angelic forces during the scanning process.

The more we practice scanning the easier it becomes. The more sensitive our palms and intuition become, the simpler it is to detect issues and patterns in a client's esoteric anatomy. We can also practice scanning on ourselves.

There are many ways to scan the esoteric anatomy. A few examples are listed below. Try one or all and see what works best for you.

1. Have the client lie face up (supine) or face down (prone). Use one or both hands. Begin the reading at the feet. Hands should be three to six inches from the client's physical body to ensure we are scanning the Body of Yetzirah (emotional body).
2. Allow the ohrim to guide the scanning process. Raise or lower the palms if the ohrim is needed more elsewhere or if we are attempting to gage information from another part of the esoteric anatomy. Staying within the Body of Yetzirah and working with the sephirot located there is a flexible guideline.
3. When scanning the front of a client's body we begin at the Sephirah of Malchut located at the feet. We move our palms up to their knees (Netzach and Hod), pelvis (Yesod), abdomen (Tipheret), arms (Gevurah and Chesed), left and right of head (Binah and Chochmah) and above their head (Keter). Then reverse from head to toes. We may stop in areas of interest to

offer ohrim or better assess what is going on within the energy. Our movements should be slow.
4. Sense how the client's energy field presents itself. Be in the moment with them. Relay information we receive from the reading to the client if it feels right to do so. Verbal exchanges lead to a deeper level of communication around the healing process.

It is not uncommon for a client to cry during a session. Let the client know that it is normal if it happens. They are releasing blocked energy. That energy may bring with it a memory, pain, a feeling or grief. Guide the client to the present moment. Honor the healing process. Let them know that once the blocked energy flows it will transform into what it is intended to be.

Not everyone is ready to experience the depth of what is held in the esoteric anatomy. We may try to avoid the pain of a blocked emotion. Unfortunately, the pain rarely disappears if it isn't felt or doesn't move. If a client does not want to continue to experience the flow of energy do not force them. It may be enough for them to know that a block is there and will move when they are ready.

If a client is receiving a KST treatment then they are ready for healing on some level. Once we process an energy block with them, they will not have to go through the pain held in that area again, as long as the incident that created the block is not repeated. The lesson of that experience will cause a transformation. After a healing it is important to continue to take right action on all levels in order to maintain a healthy energy flow in the esoteric anatomy.

As energy begins to flow during a session, our esoteric anatomy will quicken. This means the frequency will match the healthier and higher frequency of the ohrim. In this case, to feel is to heal. It is normal. If we are able to feel our pain and let it go it can transform into the next level of learning. Allow blocked energy to transform the way a caterpillar becomes a butterfly.

Part II

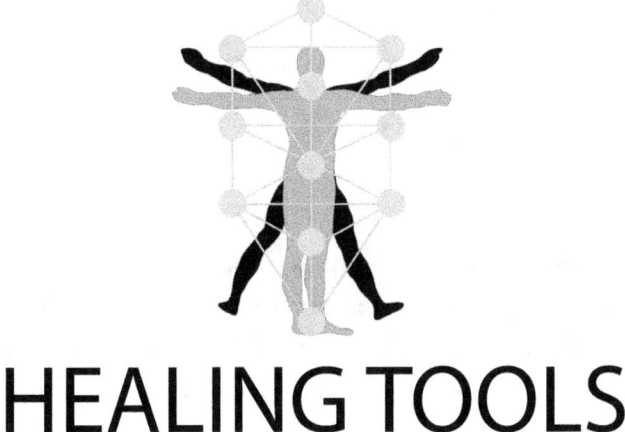

HEALING TOOLS

CHAPTER 9

Kavana

KAVANA MEANS INTENTION. As KST practitioners we are conscious of our intentions as kavana. During treatment sessions we ask what our client's kavana is for their session. Then, we hold space for that kavana during the treatment. We always have our client's highest good in mind as part of their kavana.

There are numerous healing techniques in KSTechnique® that help us to amplify kavana. There are techniques for potential imbalance of mind, body, spirit, all levels of energy and personal struggles. Learning to work with these techniques begins with getting to know the basics.

Our body is made of energy. This is the esoteric aspect of our anatomy. Learning the structure and types of energy that make up our body helps us to better understand ourselves and our client's. Understanding the esoteric physiology of the body helps us understand interaction of processes of the esoteric anatomy. Once the esoteric anatomy and physiology are understood we will have a stable framework to incorporate additional KST techniques and healing tools in the treatment space.

If we know very little about the esoteric anatomy and physiology, we can still do this work. We keep the sessions simple, and may not utilize as many healing tools. Assessing kavana is incorporated regardless of knowledge level. When a client tells us their kavana for the session, they are effectively making it a conscious intention. This is the key that allows the ohrim to flow into the space and interact with the wisdom of the client's body.

There is an ancient story about the Japanese tea ceremony. At the beginning the student learns that the tea pot is simply a tea pot. Upon further instruction the student learns the mysteries of the tea pot and the tea ceremony. Through the complexity of the ceremony the student learns the mysteries of the universe. At times the profound awareness needed to perform the tea ceremony is complicated. Once the student masters the tea ceremony the tea pot is, once again, just a tea pot.

KSTechnique® can be as simple as the first or last day of learning the tea ceremony. To keep it simple we get centered with our kavana and allow the ohrim to flow so that healing can take place. So why learn more? We study and practice in order to be an active participant in the healing process.

HOLDING SPACE

To hold space means to be fully present while observing from a place of neutrality. During a KST treatment, holding space means to be fully aware while remaining neutral to a treatment outcome. We act as a neutral catalyst for the ohrim during the healing process. When we find ourselves guiding, wanting or expecting something to happen during a session we will still be in integrity as long as we attempt to remain as neutral as possible.

As long as our kavana is for our client's highest good then even a slip into ego consciousness will be a part of the healing process. For instance, as an energy block begins to quicken in our client it may flow through our energy field. If we have a similar block in our field, we may get triggered into our own healing crises. When we are aware of our issues, we accept a healing crisis as an opportunity for our energy field to move and heal and do not attach to the triggered energy. We remain neutral and observe the movement of energy just as we observe a KST session.

Allow awareness to exist and the energy to flow through. The energy will go to where it needs to go to transform. If we don't have blocks within us that mirror our client's trauma, the energy will flow through us and we will not experience a healing crisis. With experience our capacity for empathy increases. We are able to feel our client's grief flow through us without the need to attach or judge it.

Hold space with the client in the present moment of esoteric transition and transformation. If our client can feel the grief without attachment, it will still transform. They do not need to know where it came from. Suppressing the movement of energy is what results in the energy block remaining where it was or shifting to a more rigid place in an attempt to stop movement in the future. Allow the energy to move and become what it is meant to be. The light of the ohrim will flow into the space to facilitate this process of healing.

Two additional techniques help to keep us neutral in a session. The first is to connect with tipheret consciousness. The second is to ground ourselves through malchut consciousness.

Tipheret is the central sephirot of ZA (Zeir Anpin) found in our solar plexus. It is where our personal power can be accessed. There is a calm feeling of peace and stillness when Tipheret is in balance. Remaining still within our center point of Tipheret is an important technique when we find ourselves questioning ourselves.

Grounding ourselves during and after sessions is important. A technique to help tether us is to visualize roots growing from the Sephirah of Malchut within us. Watch our roots descend into the Earth. Allow unwanted energy to descend through our roots and into the Earth. Remember that our negative energy is food for the Earth. The Earth welcomes our energy and transforms the negative energy into a nurturing golden light. Allow that light to ascend up through our roots and into our body to nourish us. Feel grounded and supported. This is malchut consciousness. Repeat as much as is needed to clear your body. If nature is accessible, connect bare feet and hands with the dirt. Lay down with your spine on the ground. Really feel the Earth and your connection with it.

What is the Space we are Holding?

Attempts to define space have preoccupied us throughout human history. Until recently we thought that matter, energy and space were separate. Today it appears they may not be as different as we thought.

In ancient Greece atoms were the original building blocks of creation. In 442BC, Democritus said atoms were indivisible and indestructible. Today we know that the atom is at least ninety-nine percent empty space. As we continue to break down the particles that make an atom we discover that they are also made up of mostly empty space. Below the Plank scale the laws of particle physics give way to thinking of matter as energy, quantum wave patterns or strings of energy. All of these particles and energy have their own frequency. We also have our own frequency within this orchestra of life.

We interact with physical matter as reality rather than an energy of space and illusion in order to maintain a productive level of functioning in our life. Stay grounded in the mundane day-to-day but remember that matter is both particle, energy and space. It is mate-ve-lo-mate. This is the beginning of a stable spiritual life. These truths exist and can coexist. Live life with this knowledge in order to expand awareness. We know that things are solid and are not solid at the same time.

Our body is solid. But it's underlying nature is energy. Our physical body is a layer of energy that moves at a slower frequency than our more subtle bodies of energy. In KST our physical body of energy is called the Body of Asiyah. It encompasses both matter and energy as one.

The element of earth contains all of the other elements and supports them. Space as the element of aether is what contains the other elements as potential. If earth is a physical particle then aether is its true nature as the space that contains matter.

When we hold space in the treatment room, we can imagine it as aether holding the universe. In that moment we mirror the microcosm of a KST treatment with the macrocosm of the universe. This helps us to master the art of holding space.

UNCONDITIONAL LOVE

OUR GREATEST HEALING TOOL is unconditional love. This is not love in the traditional sense. It is an ancient kabbalistic love that blends the giving of the Sephirah of Chesed with the restriction of the Sephirah of Gevurah. This creates the balanced love found in the Sephirah of Tipheret between them.

Chesed is love as modern western culture defines love. It is giving as a form of love. But giving without end drains us. It can easily turn us into a human doormat. That kind of love doesn't necessarily do the receiver any good. Receiving Chesed without earning it will result in our taking it for granted. We need to feel as though we earned what we were given. We need to be a worthy or stable vessel to contain what is received.

Unconditional love requires the giving of Chesed be balanced with the boundaries and restriction of Gevurah. Unconditional love has the same frequency as the ohrim. It is balance in accordance with divine purpose. It is a mirror of the neutral space we experience in a treatment session. Neutrality allows our client to process at their own pace, with their own innate wisdom. We support their process.

ENERGY HOLDS AND TREATMENT OPTIONS

AN ENERGY HOLD IS the practice of placing hands on designated points of the body or energy field. Our hands can be on or off of the body. They can be done while the client rests on a massage table, sits in a massage chair with you standing beside them, while both the client and we are seated in separate chairs or at a distance. In distance healing we do not have to be in physical proximity to the client.

How to hold that which is beyond the physical senses?

Doing an energy hold with a laying on of hands does not require belief, intention or contemplation. The physical body is over two-thirds water with currents of electricity coursing throughout it. We are human batteries. We need only do an energy hold that matches the polarity of our client in order to facilitate the exchange and flow of energy.

If a client's sephirot are all in balance we can still perform an energy hold. Our work goes beyond time and space. The ohrim may be needed for another time. We make a kavana to send ohrim to the past or future as well as the eternal now. A client's treatment request means there is a purpose for it. The treatment can be as simple as holding space for overall healing. Or we can cradle their feet to further ground the balanced sephirot.

If we are working with healing tools, we have two options. We can assess which sephirah/sephirot are out of balance and use the healing tool designated for that sephirah/sephirot. We can also ask the client what their favorite one is. For instance, if we use chromotherapy (light therapy) we ask what their favorite color is and use it. For essential oils we have them smell the various oils and pick which one resonates with them in the moment. We then coordinate the element associated with the chosen color or essential oil and do the designated energy holds for that element. Being flexible in order to accommodate client needs is key for a successful session.

Another technique is to hold kavana with a client during meditation. Adding an aether cradle at their head to facilitate the energy flow from the Sephirah of Keter will help the client relax during their mediation.

Why are facilitators of healing needed if all we are doing is remaining neutral to a treatment outcome? And why all of these healing tools? An analogy would be using an insulated copper wire instead of an uninsulated iron wire in our home. Both will facilitate the transfer of energy in a direct pathway. However, the copper will conduct energy more quickly and efficiently. In KSTechnique, the insulation is the healing kavana of the KST practitioner and the copper is holding space with a neutral and loving belief system.

It is important to explore various paths and decide which one works best for us. All true paths work with the same healing energy and intentions. It is up to us as conscious conduits and co-creators to embrace that which works best with our own individual human battery, soul, consciousness and desire.

Astrology and the Energy Hold

Astrology studies the placement, movement and relative positions of stars and other celestial objects and connects that information to human and earthly events. The western zodiac includes twelve characters in the sky. These personas are made out of a collection of stars that are connected from our perspective. Each sign has an associated body part, element, temperament and purpose.

During a KST session, it is helpful to know what the client's astrological sign is. Knowing which part of the body the astrological sign coordinates with determines the client's critical or sensitive points in both their body and mind.

Zodiac signs, elements and energy holds are the same in KSTechnique, Kabbalah and the Vedas. This is due to the exchange of information between the East Indian Vedas and the Kabbalah of ancient Mesopotamia.

Later, the astrology between the Vedas and Kabbalah diverged. The Vedas became an equally transcendent albeit different system of astrology called Jotish. But the similarities are much greater than the differences for the purposes of KSTechnique. For instance, both kabbalistic astrology and Jotish are based on sidereal astrology, whereby celestial interpretations change with the shifts of our constellations. Non kabbalistic western astrology works on a fixed system and thus is not as accurate at times.

In Kabbalah, Ayurveda and KSTechnique, the twelve signs of the zodiac correspond to different parts of the body. By knowing which astrological sign corresponds to which body part we are able to do a more detailed assessment and treatment plan for our clients. Astrology makes a wonderful healing tool.

The esoteric anatomy and the astrological signs are interwoven. Once these systems are memorized we can see the repetition of patterns that exist in them. It is a spectacular kaleidoscope of creative expression. Begin by memorizing which astrological signs go with which body part one by one.

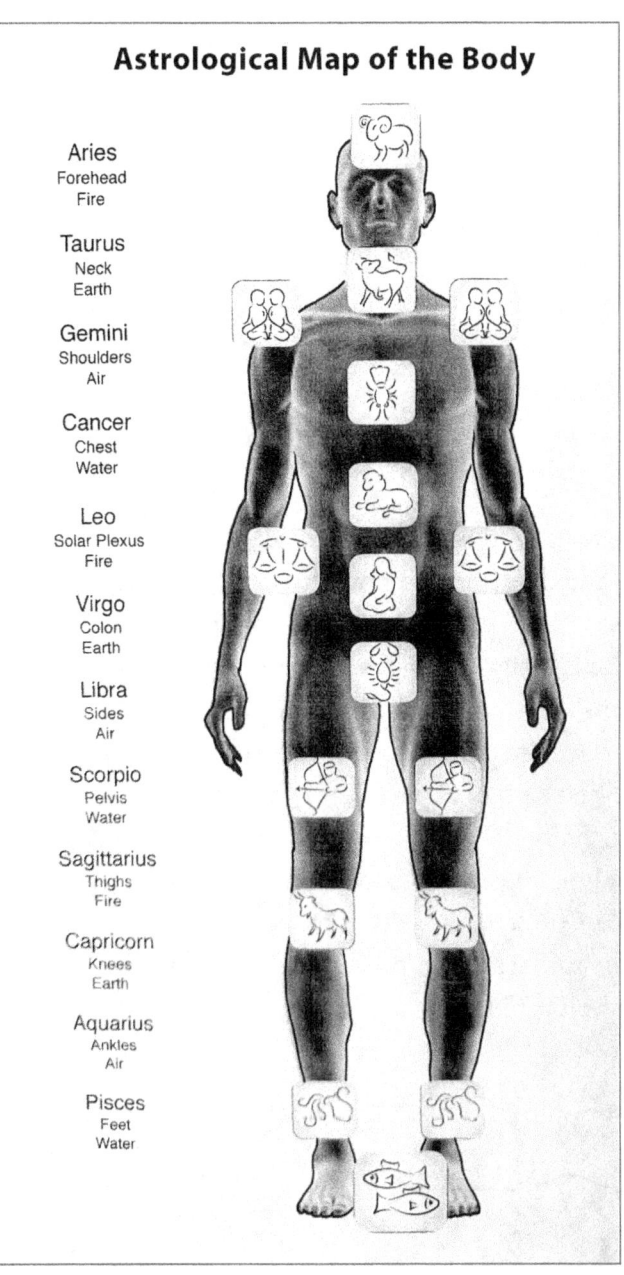

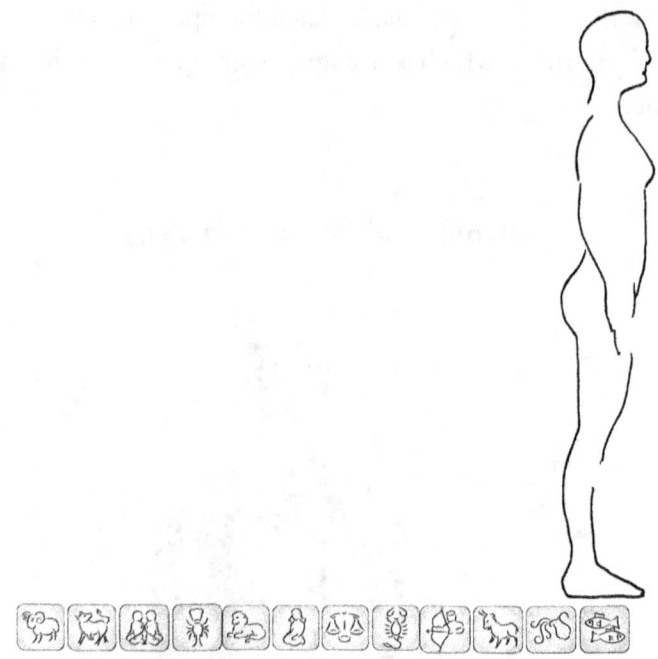

Try this visualization to help memorize the connection between the zodiac and a body. Visualize how the twelve constellations are placed across the sky. Now picture a person standing at the right end of the zodiac at the last sign of Pisces. Have the person face away from the constellations as though they are about to lay down on them.

Finally, have the person lay down with their feet at Pisces and their head at the first sign of Aries. That is how the astrological signs coordinate with the body. The elements and constitutions associated with the zodiac signs line up with our body. They mirror the parts of the body they come in contact with. For instance, the fiery Aries is associated with the forehead where the symbol of Shin, or Fire Constitution in the body is located.

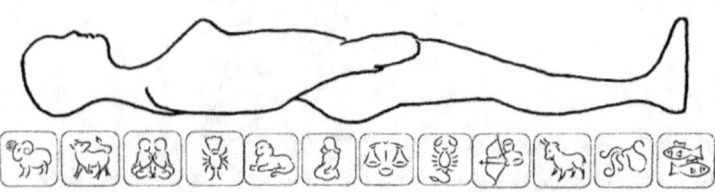

Which Energy Holds and Elements?

Energy holds are a key part of a KST treatment. Healing tools are optional but energy holds are constant. They help balance the client. There are different energy hold protocols for each element. Each element is associated with a sephirah or set of sephirot.

The right column of the ToL *(Refer back to the ToL / Ten Sephirot illustration in Chapter 2)* is made up of the Sephirot of Netzach, Chesed and Chochmah, which are associated with the water element. The left column of the ToL is made up of the Sephirot of Hod, Gevurah and Binah, which are associated with the fire element. The central column of the ToL finds Malchut at the bottom, which is associated with the element of earth. Above Malchut is Yesod and Tipheret, which are associated with the element of air. At the top of the central column of the ToL we find Keter, which is associated with the element of aether.

How Does Energy Feel?

How do we hold energy? It is not accessible to our physical senses. But it can be! There are two ways to feel energy. The first is to sense the energy naturally. The second is simply to learn that energy exists.

KST promotes exercises that will help the practitioner experience energy. Sometimes this occurs right away. Other times it takes doing many treatments to start to feel it. Either way an energy protocol will succeed if done correctly. We don't have to believe that healing energy exists. It simply exists.

One way to begin to sense energy is to hold our hands about a foot apart for about thirty to sixty-seconds. Slowly bring the hands closer and closer toward each other. We slowly shift our hands as though we are holding a ball of energy. As our hands get to be within a few inches of each other it will feel as though there is a tangible sensation pushing them apart. Once we reach that point of resistance, we continue to experiment by moving our hands both toward and away from each other. Focus on the sensations. We blur our vision as we look at our hands. Become aware of the energy that is between them. This is the energy that exists around all things.

WHAT MAKES A HEALER?

WE ARE ALL HEALERS. Anyone can learn to heal. The ability to heal comes more naturally to some. It is the same as someone having 20/20 vision and another person having 20/30 vision. They both have the ability to see. The latter will need to use glasses in order to have the same ability to see as the person with 20/20 vision. A person with natural healing ability is like the person with 20/20 vision. The natural healer can perform healing protocols without healing tools. But without training and practice even the natural healer may not be affective.

Healing is one percent talent and ninety-nine percent practice. Some of us may be lucky and have five or even twenty percent of the ability easily accessible to us. The question is, will we take it for granted since it comes so easily to us or will we work to truly develop our talents?

Environment plays a key role in the development of a healer. If we are naturally good at healing and have a guardian who is a holistic therapist our environment may compel us to focus, study and identify with being a holistic minded person. From the outside it may appear that we were just naturally born that way.

The more we practice correctly the more our abilities will bloom. Healing is as innate to our body as any of our other senses. Our connection with this healing ability is embedded in our DNA. We need only realize it. Focus, study, practice and learn and our healing potential will unfold.

Be diligent in the art of healing. Allow the senses to perceive beyond physical constraints. There are as many ways to sense the energy field as there are healers. Some healers will see energy, others will smell, hear, feel or intuit energy and the esoteric anatomy. Once we know where our talents lie in sensing energy we can recognize and utilize the information in our practice.

At times we may sense our client's overall esoteric anatomy and other times just a portion of the information may come. This can occur with any of the senses. Each treatment is unique and each one has its purpose. Allow the treatment's meaning to unfold as it is meant to.

Professional Boundaries

As healers we want to give of ourselves. But we need to maintain boundaries in order to be effective. This means knowing ourselves and our limits. We need to know how the Sephirot of Chesed and Gevurah balance in our center of Tipheret as unconditional love. It also means knowing the laws within the jurisdiction we live and work in. These boundaries will determine how to apply KST protocols in effective ways.

Energy holds are key to a KST treatment protocol. They can be done with our hands on or off of the body depending on client need and licensing requirements within our jurisdiction. For instance, if we are doing a body treatment, we may need a massage license to do a hands-on treatment. If we are a psychotherapist, we may choose to do an energy hold from across the room or work in conjunction with a licensed bodyworker.

Most KST practitioners without other licenses may choose to work with people on a massage table. In these cases, the client is fully clothed at all times. When doing an energy hold off of the body make sure hands are one inch to one foot off of the body if you are working with the Body of Yetzirah (emotional body). If we are placing our hands on the physical, we make sure our hands are relaxed with gentle pressure on the client's contact points. Avoid any areas that are deemed private by our society and for our client. Client privacy is determined by both the law and client comfort. We assess a client's need of additional privacy with the use of verbal and written intake forms.

During a treatment we adjust certain contact points. For instance, when working on the back of the body, we place our hand on the lower sacrum when working on the Sephirot of Malchut rather than on the anus. For the Heart of Binah, we place our hand on the upper decollete to avoid breast tissue. Always be considerate of a client's personal space and person.

Maintain healthy professional boundaries and our client's benefit. Boundaries help create a healthy and nurturing environment. We will be less likely to unintentionally recreate the feeling of abuse with those who have previously experienced it. We will mitigate issues of transference or counter-transference so the client or practitioner does not project their issues unto each other. We are here to heal and sometimes healing means relying on Gevurah for good judgment and boundaries in order to facilitate the flow of the ohrim.

Chapter 10

Protocols

THERE ARE AS MANY PROTOCOLS as there are grains of sand. KST protocols are blueprints for healing. They give a practitioner guidance within the infinite potential of the ohrim. KST protocols work in synergy with our practice to maximize a therapeutic potential. They are a supportive healing tool but not an absolute. They provide a structure for the ultimate truth to express itself but are not the ultimate truth.

KST protocols can vary depending on the treatment setting. In the spa, a treatment may include essential oils, chromotherapy, a foot wrap, energy work and bodywork. A psychotherapy session could include verbal and written assessments, processing and distance healing.

There are a few key elements that underly all KST protocols. They include maintaining neutral kavana, assessment, reading the ToL, treatment application, processing and closure. The protocols that follow are suggestive frameworks. To really perform a protocol correctly requires training. Please only experiment with these protocols after you have been trained by a KST professional and have been trained in your own area of expertise. Do not do any treatment that is outside of your scope of practice.

PROCEDURE

NEUTRAL KAVANA IS THE INTENTION we bring into each treatment. We set the room as a sacred space. We become a conduit for the ohrim by embracing the correct kavana. Remain in a neutral and unconditionally loving space while acting as a conduit for the ohrim during each treatment. This enables the ohrim to express itself in a perfect way for our clients. The result is not up to us. The definition and method of kavana was covered more thoroughly in chapter nine.

During the client intake, ask if they have an intention or kavana for their session. It is empowering for a client to recognize the kavana that brought them to their session. It is important for the practitioner to hear the client's kavana. It helps us to focus on what the client wants to work on. A client's kavana can be physical, emotional or spiritual in nature.

As a practitioner, a mate-ve-lo-mate experience is to be both an active and passive participant in the treatment process. Being an active participant requires knowledge and experience. Being a passive practitioner means we are receptive to the flow of the ohrim and are unattached to the treatment outcome. Being prepared and doing a thorough intake with our client ensures we can be of optimal help for them.

Following the intake, we read the ToL for our client. This can be done whether the client is physically present or not. The client may be on a massage table, sitting, standing or in a different location. The reading may be done with a pendulum, hand or intuition. The key is to tune into the ToL and listen for its expression.

The sephirot are read from below to above: from Malchut to Keter. We start from our physical perspective and ascend the ToL. Tell the client what is being read in each sephirah. Ask if the information resonates with them. Dialogue helps to move energy. The sephirotic script in the section titled, "Sephirotic Script," is a good blueprint to use during this reading.

After the ToL reading our focus shifts to how energy is transforming during the treatment. Processing refers to this movement of energy. Energy movements occur on a physical, emotional or spiritual level.

If performing a service at a spa, the client may want to express what they are experiencing or they may be silent. In a psychotherapeutic setting the client will ideally focus on verbal processing, or other creative expression such as drawing or movement.

We process through verbal and creative methods with clients to the extent that we are trained. For instance, a bodyworker will be able to help someone process physically more than a psychotherapist. Therapeutic partnerships between psychotherapists and bodyworkers is one way to attend to a client's needs more fully.

As a session begins to come to an end, create a sense of closure for your client. This can be done by reviewing the session as a synopsis. Ask if there is anything more the client needs to feel like the session is complete. If the client has been silent or has fallen asleep during a session feel free to gently wake them. If a question or continued symptom persists feel free to answer or accommodate it. The client's request should value the therapeutic intention.

Closure is to the end of the session as setting the correct kavana is to the beginning of it. As the Sefer Yetzirah says, "the end is embedded in the beginning, and their beginning in their end."[26] Closure of one treatment leads to another level of healing and experience.

Remembering RT

RT (Ruah Technique) is the breathing technique that was explored in chapter three. Perform RT prior to doing a KSTechnique® protocol. We center ourselves as we breathe. Inhale ohrim and imagine it as the air that we breathe and the blood that distributes it throughout our body.

Basic RT protocol for individual or group practice:
1. Sit or stand comfortably.
2. Guide your consciousness to your breath.
3. Relax your jaw.
4. Quiet your mind.
5. Focus on your breath.

6. On the in-hale, constrict your throat until you hear a wind tunnel-like sound. Continue breathing in with that sound for the full inhalation.
7. Hold the breath until you need to release it.
8. Produce the same wind tunnel-like sound on the exhale. Make sure the exhale is longer than the inhale. Completely empty the contents of your lungs and abdomen.
9. Hold the breath until you need to inhale.
10. Repeat cycle on inhale.
11. Perform RT for a few minutes in the morning and a few minutes in the evening preferably just prior to meditation.

RT protocol for energy clearing:
1. Sit or stand comfortably.
2. Guide your consciousness to your breath.
3. Relax your jaw.
4. Quiet your mind.
5. Imagine a white light above you. Allow that light to enter through the crown of your head as you slowly inhale while making the wind tunnel sound. Fill your throat, chest and belly with a conscious breath. Hold the breath as long as is comfortable. Release.
6. On the exhale imagine the white light descending with your breath, down you head, neck, torso and continuing down your legs and through your feet. Connect with the earth and allow the light to reach further into the depths of the earth. Make sure the ex-hale is longer than the inhale.
7. Imagine the white light in the earth transforming into a golden light. Hold the exhale as long as is comfortable.
8. Slowly in-hale. See that gold light flow to your feet, up through your legs, torso, neck and head. Connect with the wind tunnel sound as you inhale. Allow you breath and the golden light of the earth to nurture and fill your being as it connects with the white light above.

9. Hold the breath until you need to release it.
10. Repeat.

Practicing RT outside the treatment setting is highly recommended. Use it whenever you need to clear your body of an imbalance of energy. The white light is the pure light of the ohrim that brings all that needs to be transformed within you to the earth.

Our negativity is food for the earth just as our carbon dioxide is life sustaining for a plant. The earth has the ability to utilize our negativity and transform it into a healing and protective golden light that gifts us with health and help.

INTRODUCTION TO THE SEPHIROTIC SCRIPT

KNOWING THE BASIC CHARACTERISTICS OF EACH SEPHIRAH is helpful during a KST reading. Memorizing the details of each of the sephirah listed in the sephirotic script below will enable us to do a solid ToL reading for our client.

For instance, If a client is changing careers our reading of the Sephirah of Malchut may show confusion. This is because Malchut is associated with grounding and stability around areas of survival. This holds true whether the new career is a positive or negative move.

All change creates stress in the body. We find a center point of balance to get through a challenging time. Air is the neutral force that decides between the left side of fire and ice and right side of water. Likewise, change is the neutral force which can be either positive or negative. It is up to us to channel our experience of stress in a constructive way. We guide our clients to choose a positive way to approach their stress.

Script for Reading of Sephirot

This section contains a sephirotic script. It contains a few details about each of the sephirah being read during a KST treatment. Some practitioners memorize the script while others read it from a sheet of paper or use sephirah placement cards.

Memorizing sephirotic details and placements might seem overwhelming at first. To manage the task, perform an imaginary reading twice per day for three weeks. For instance, if we are using a pendulum, hold the pendulum over the imagined area being read. Have the sephirot script in the other hand and read from it, then, move the pendulum to the next sephirah and read the next description. Do this until the reading is complete. After three weeks you will have memorized the script. It is not magic. It's simply neural connections growing in our brain as a result of repetition.

In class, we place laminated representations of the sephirot on the areas we read. One side of the laminates has a picture of the ToL with the associated sephirah highlighted. Put this side of the laminate facing upward. The other side of the laminate has the script written on it. Pick up the laminated circle of the sephirah being assessed. Then read the description on the laminate while holding the pendulum over the sephirah on the client's body. Look and describe what the pendulum is doing. Then, place the laminate back with the ToL facing up.

Trying to remember details about each sephirah during a treatment can be stressful. Memorizing the script can free our mind of this stress. We can focus on the treatment process and the flow of the ohrim. Being stress free and present during the healing process is like watching the meaning of the universe unfold.

We step out of your own way and allow the universal healing energy of the ohrim to guide us.

Example of Script for Reading Front and Back of Body

Malchut, first sephirah: Front (pendulum above the center of feet) Back (pendulum below coccyx)
- Contains all colors of the rainbow
- Element of earth or dust

It's about grounding, stability in the world, survival and getting rid of waste.

Yesod, second sephirah: Front (pendulum above pelvis) Back (pendulum over low back)
- Sephirah of foundation
- Color of purple or indigo
- Element of air

It's about sensuality, creativity, interpersonal connections.

Hod, third sephirah: Front (pendulum above left knee) Back (pendulum over left kidney) Sephirah of splendor.
- Color of orange
- Element of fire

It's about conscious intellect, individual personality and rational. It's also our capacity for empathy.

Netzach, fourth sephirah: Front (pendulum above right knee) Back (pendulum over right kidney)
- Sephirah of victory
- Color of green
- Element of water

It's about the unconscious which controls so much of our lives. Our instinctual nature.

Tipheret, fifth sephirah: Front (pendulum above solar plexus) Back (pendulum over mid back / thoracic)
- Sephirah of beauty
- Color of light yellow or pink
- Element of air... Yet it contains all of the elements except for earth.

It's about unification and stillness. It's the balance point for all aspects of our true nature. Our sense of self and personal power.

Gevurah, sixth sephirah: Front (pendulum above the left arm) Back (pendulum above left arm)

- Sephirah of restraint
- Color of red
- Element of fire

It's about personal boundaries. Our ability to discern, maintain objectivity when judging situations or people.

Chesed, seventh sephirah: Front (pendulum above right arm); Back (pendulum above right arm)
- Sephirah of love
- Color of blue
- Element of water

It's the blueprint for our feelings around love. It's our desire to give unconditionally.

Binah, eighth sephirah: Front (pendulum on left side of head in level I); Back (pendulum on left side of head in level I)
- Sephirah of understanding
- Color of black or crimson
- Element of fire

It's the heart mind, the center of emotional connection and true understanding.

Chochmah, ninth sephirah: Front (pendulum on right side of head in level I); Back (pendulum on right side of head in level I)
- Sephirah of wisdom
- Color of soft blue or grey
- Element of water

It's about expansion, limitless wisdom, intellect & linear thinking.

Keter, tenth sephirah: Front (pendulum above the crown of the head in level I); Back (pendulum above the back of head in level I)
- Crown sephirah
- Color of white
- Element of aether

It's about our connection with our higher self. About finding our true path in this life.

TREATMENT PROTOCOLS

Massage Table Protocol

Horizontal client positioning is perfect for KST practitioners, bodyworkers and estheticians. It is an effective way to read and balance the ToL in the body. By allowing access to the circumference of the client's body, we can conduct a reading and treatment with ease. The client should be clothed at all times during a KST treatment. Exceptions to the clothing rule include a KST treatment being done by a licensed therapist in a spa, therapeutic bodywork or medical setting. In these cases, attention should be on legal requirements in our jurisdiction and appropriate draping techniques.

From a psychological perspective, when a client is horizontal on a massage table and the therapist is vertical the therapist will be perceived to be in a power position. Depending on the client's previous life experiences this may or may not present an issue. For instance, if the client is a regular spa goer, resting on a massage table triggers relaxation. However, if the client is new to healing or spa modalities, they may feel a sense of unwelcome vulnerability. As practitioners we are sensitive to our client's well-being.

When an issue does arise, either positive or negative, allow it to be a part of the therapeutic session. If the client wants to stop the session at any time, stop. If they want to breathe through and explore a therapeutic occurrence, continue. Allow tears to flow as easily as laughter, chatter or silence. By honoring where our client is at each moment we help create a safe place for healing to occur.

Example of Massage Table Protocol:
1. Explain treatment.
2. Inquire verbally about client kavana.
3. Perform assessment. This can be a review of a written intake form, pulse testing, essential oil preferences or other.
4. Ask client to remove their shoes and lay supine on the massage or medical table.

5. Place bolster under knees and neck pillow under the neck and head.
6. Spray Essence Spray (optional).
7. Body Alignment Adjustments (optional).
8. Four gates on ankles and wrists (optional).
9. Read sephirot with pendulum or hand beginning at Malchut and ending with Keter.
10. Ask which sephirah or sephirot the client wants to work on.
11. Perform energy holds associated with chosen sephirah or sephirot.
12. Remove bolster and neck and head pillow.
13. Have guest turn prone.
14. Place bolster under ankles for guest comfort.
15. Four gates (optional.
16. Perform energy holds associated with the sephirah being worked on.
17. Energy holds on occiput and sacrum (optional).
18. Sephirah spray (optional).
19. Place guest's shoes on side of table.
20. Closure.

Seated Protocol

Both client and practitioner can be seated during a KST session. If the client is seated and the therapist is standing the same principles from the previous section (massage table protocol) apply.

When the KST practitioner and client are seated in separated chairs the session becomes easily incorporated into psychotherapeutic modalities. This method is appropriate for psychologists, psychotherapists, physicians and KST practitioners.

The session includes verbal and written assessments, distance reading, verbal evaluation and processing, treatment and closure. Treatment for these sessions revolve around verbal exchange, meditation or distance healing.

Example of Seated Protocol:
1. Intake.
2. Ask for client kavana.
3. Have client sit comfortably in a chair, knees in front and both feet flat on the ground before them. Their legs are in a 45-degree angle. Arms and hands rest on top of their respective legs
4. Guide client in a few RT breaths.
5. Read sephirot on front of the body with pendulum or hand beginning at Malchut and ending with Keter. Discuss results with client.
6. Ask which sephirah client would like to work on.
7. Perform energy holds for that sephirah both on front and back of body using visualization.
8. Closure.

Standing Protocol

Standing is an art form. Our stance determines so much about how we feel and how energy flows in our body. Practicing a healthy stance can help us remain centered in our practice. Learning to read our stance can offer valuable information as to what might be troubling us. For instance, if we are emotionally withdrawn our shoulders may collapse around our heart and rib cage. This will create slowing of energy in our body and a barrier toward others. Pressing our shoulders down and away from our ears while expanding them outward and back helps release the flow of energy.

Assessing another person's stance is also a valuable assessment tool to use with our clients. During a KST treatment a client's stance is assessed. This can be done as part of another protocol or as a treatment by itself. Our client's stance tells us a lot about them and where they are in the moment. When a client's stance is shifted to a healthier one as part of a treatment it allows the energy to flow. Opening to that flow can facilitate healing.

Once we learn the meaning of different stances, we can begin to assess which sephirah may be out of balance prior to a ToL reading. Adjusting a client's stance so that energy flows better may be done prior to or following a reading. When we do feel the need to adjust a client's stance we do so gently and therapeutically. These adjustments can be done while the client is standing or while they are resting on a massage table.

A general guideline for proper stance requires that both feet face front, hip width apart, with knees slightly bent. Sacrum and shoulders are horizontal to each other, arms and hands are relaxed by the sides. Shoulders should be relaxed, down and back away from the ears. Neck has a slight curve but head stands above the torso. Breathing should be slow, conscious and not forced. The breath will fill the chest and abdomen. Ask how the client feels in the moment. Do they experience any shifts of energy, comfort or discomfort? If so, why?

As practitioners it is important for us to adjust our stance as a regular part of our therapeutic practice. Doing the same for a client can bring shifts and awareness necessary for healing and growth.

Example of Standing Protocol:

When conducting a ToL reading while the client is standing, stand beside the client and hold the pendulum a few inches to a foot away from the sephirah placement on the body. Our hands will be higher than the sephirah being read so the chain of the pendulum has enough length to swing properly. The pendant part of the pendulum will be in direct contact with the sephirah's energy center.

1. Intake.
2. Inquire about client's kavana for session.
3. Read sephirot on front or back of body with pendulum beginning at Malchut and ending with Keter.
4. Ask which sephirah feels like it needs to be worked on.
5. Adjust client's stance if needed. Make sure that client is standing with knees loose, feet hip width apart, pelvis in

alignment with the back and shoulders, arms comfortable by their side and head over torso.
6. Have client get in touch with the energy flow the new stance creates.
7. Discuss reading.
8. Closure.

Spa Protocol

Below is a sample spa protocol that includes pulse testing, aromatherapy, kavana assessment, medical assessment, ToL reading, bodywork, energy holds and closure. This treatment requires all therapists be licensed massage practitioners and participate in an accredited level one KSP course. Therapists who go on to do KSP level II and III are able to incorporate other techniques into this service including setting the treatment space with healing symbols and working with angelic energy. A couple of these therapists have submitted case studies that are included in chapter eighteen titled, "Case Studies."

Example of Spa Protocol:

Materials Needed: Massage table, linens, essential oils and spray, chromotherapy light, neck roll, pendulum, bolster, tuning forks, CMBr soundtrack, face cradle.
1. Explain treatment for client.
2. Inquire about client kavana for the treatment.
3. Ask about any medical issues or areas of concern.
4. Ask guest to lie supine on the massage table.
5. Leave while guest gets on the massage table.
6. Place bolster under client's knees.
7. Spray essence spray.
8. Four gates on ankles and wrists.
9. Body alignment adjustments.
10. Read ToL with pendulum.

11. Ask client which sephirah they would prefer to work on.
12. Turn chromotherapy light to color associated with sephirah being worked on.
13. Apply elemental essential oil and crystal blend associated with the sephirah being worked on.
14. Crystal placement.
15. Perform energy work sequence (from sephirot body points cheat sheet for front of body).
16. Massage front of body managing crystals as you go.
17. Remove crystals.
18. Remove bolster.
19. Ask client to turn prone while you hold the sheet covering them in a tent like fashion.
20. Apply elemental essential oil blend associated with the sephirah being worked on.
21. Crystal placement.
22. Play CMBr.
23. Perform energy work sequence (from sephirot body point cheat sheet for back of body).
24. Massage back of body adjusting crystals as needed.
25. KSH energy hold on occiput and sacrum. Release.
26. KSH energy hold with both hands on occiput. Release.
27. Sephirah spray.
28. Chime tuning forks.
29. Explain that the treatment has come to a close.
30. Place client's shoes on side of table and their robe over the sheet covering their ankles. Place water next to client's ticket if available.
31. Leave room.

KSH Protocol

KSH (Kabbalah Somatic Hold) is a protocol that works with the invisible Sephirah of Da'at. This sephirah is reviewed in greater depth in chapter sixteen titled, "Soul Traveling and Da'at."

Bodyworkers can access Da'at by holding or massaging the area around the occiput at the back of the head and neck. The occiput is the area that helps us access the unification or soul traveling experience.

KST practitioners can perform a KSH or the KS hold by following the protocol below. Psychotherapists can do KSH via distance healing using the KSH protocol as a framework. They can also work in conjunction with a bodyworker who can perform the hold. The psychotherapist can discuss the client's experience in depth afterward.

The KSH protocol is meant to help balance the Supernal Triad by bringing the ToL into harmony with the body, mind and spirit. This strengthens the vessel of the body so that it can hold more ohrim.

Example of KSH Protocol

Client is supine on a massage table. Stand beside the client and either sit in a chair or squat until your shoulders are in line with the massage table.

1. With palms up, place one hand under client's occiput and other under the sacrum. Hold kavana until you feel the client's energy begin to flow. It will feel like a pulse between your hands. Gently release the hold by drawing your hands out from under the client's body.
2. Move to the head of your client. Sit in a chair or squat so that your shoulders are in line with the massage table. Place both of your hands, palms up, under the client's shoulders. Remain there until you feel a pulse. Bring both hands together. Place them under the client's occiput until the client's head rests comfortably in both palms. Wait until you feel a pulse. Release your hands from under the client's neck.
3. Cradle the back of the client's head with your thumbs at KT and your four other fingers evenly spaced on the temporal region of the client's head. Wait to feel a pulse. Release.
4. Place one hand beneath the client's neck while your other hand rests on the client's forehead. Wait until you feel a pulse. Release.
5. Continue to hold client's forehead while you move your other

hand around their upper decollete. Avoid breast tissue. Wait until you feel a pulse. Release.

Foot Protocol

The entire body is mapped out on our feet, hands and ears. Working on the feet helps us stabilize the Sephirah of Malchut and draw stability and abundance to our lives. This treatment should only be performed by licensed bodyworkers or reflexologists.

KSTechnique® foot protocol is a compliment to any bodywork treatment. It is also a perfect way to ground the KSH protocol. This foot protocol can be a treatment by itself.

Example of Foot Protocol

To perform a protocol correctly requires training. Please only experiment with these protocols after you have been trained by a KSTechnique® professional and have been trained in your own area of expertise. Do not do any treatment that is outside of your scope of practice.

1. Place oil or lotion on clean foot using soothing strokes.
2. Kneel or sit. Use knuckles to strip plantar fascia, then heels using clasped hands. Inch fingers slowly upward along vertical lines, beginning at base of the heel and ending at the toes.
3. Use knuckles to strip lung area, then apply pressure to points along shoulder area of foot, then diaphragm, while simultaneously folding top of foot over diaphragm point.
4. Stand. Use deep, soothing, circular pressure all over the area just worked.
5. Kneel or sit. Do inching thumb pressures along pressure points. Begin with holding sacral points with one hand and doing circular movements on the heel with the other.
6. Horizontal, then lateral inching across heels.
7. Diagonal inching from mid-line of plantar fascia to medial side of foot, then from mid-line to lateral side of foot, up to the diaphragm.

Foot Reflexology Chart

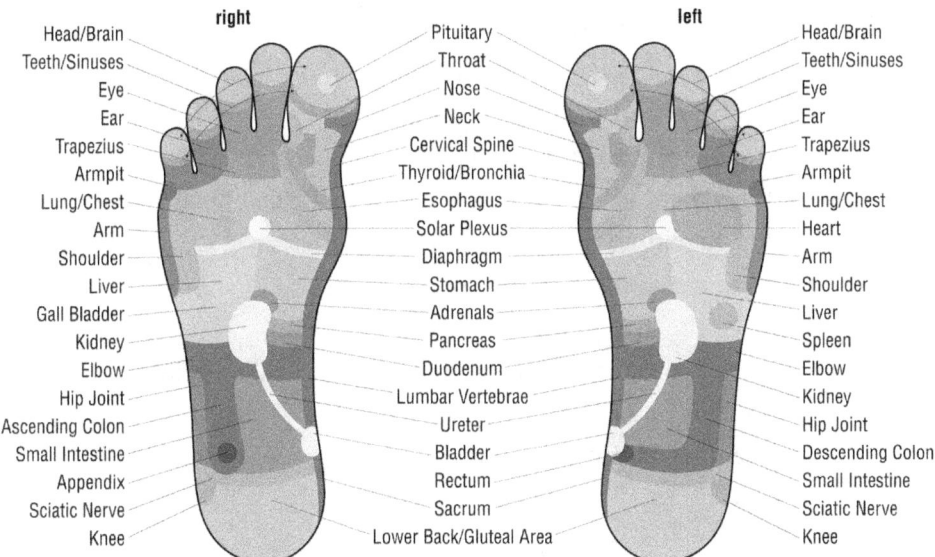

8. Perform inching movements across chest point, both horizontal and laterally.
9. Apply pressure down the five lines found between the toes on front of foot using inching movements.
10. Use deep, soothing, circular pressure massage all over area just worked beginning at top of foot near toes and ending at the ankle.
11. Perform inching movement with all four fingers across top of foot, 3x12. Hold at either end of lymph area around ankles and inch toward center, 3x.
12. Place opposite hand to client's foot (for left foot use your right hand. For right foot use your left hand). Strip upward until you reach the big toe.
13. Slowly begin inching movements up each toe. Pay careful attention to the neck and sinus points.
14. Start from the bottom portion of the heel with both hands on either side of foot, shimmy hands until you reach the toes.

Begin the same movement from both sides of the foot, starting at the heel and ending at the beginning of the toes.
15. Do a shimmy with each toe individually.
16. Perform an energy hold with one hand on bottom of foot and the other on top of foot.
17. Do the same on the other foot.
18. Once both feet have been worked, hold both feet at the same time. Massage up both feet.
19. Inch down the spinal points, 3x.
20. Inch down the arm points, 3x.
21. Do an energy hold at sciatic point, solar plexus, heart and sinus points.
22. Slowly remove hands from feet.

Chapter 11

Esoteric Anatomy

All that He had made—all in one totality, above and below.[27]
— *Zohar,* Daniel C. Matt

BY LOOKING OUTWARD into the vastness of creation we begin to view the macrocosm of our inner truth. By looking within, these mysteries unfold until we see our bodies as a blueprint of the olamot worlds.

Olamot refers to the five worlds that make up our universe.

Sephirot, meaning "enumerations," refers to the ten attributes that make up creation.

The esoteric anatomy of our body is mirrored within the five olamot worlds and the sephirot that make up all of creation. As such, our body is merely a microcosm of the macrocosm around us. The process of creation describes how this came to be. Kabbalah and cosmology explore this process in different ways that ultimately mean the same thing. It is this process of creation and universal structure that offers a blueprint for us to follow in our quest for understanding and healing.

When we look outward with the tool of cosmology, we see how the universe originated as pure light. The four forces of physics: the strong nuclear force, the weak nuclear force, electromagnetism and gravity, did not even exist yet. There was only pure light and heat. As creation cooled, the light retreated, the natural forces began to manifest and energy became particles. Thus did matter come from energy and light, the resonance of which exists today in the cosmic microwave background radiation, or CMBr. We will explore this more thoroughly in chapter sixteen, "Soul Traveling." The CMBr is the cooled remnant of the hot Big Bang. The Big Bang took place in complete silence but, as the universe expanded, sound waves were able to grow. Thus did sound or the cosmic word, usher in the age of the physical.

According to Kabbalah, prior to creation only Ein Sof existed. This existence was beyond time and space and beyond our physical ability to comprehend it. When creation was first initiated, there was only a manifestation of Ein Sof as a reflected whisper of the ultimate truth. It took form as pure light and tohu (chaos). This mirrors the quantum state prior to the Big Bang. In order for there to be a world, the infinite light had to be removed, otherwise there would have been no room for creation as we understand it. The act of tzimtzum (the removal as contraction of light) enabled the creative process of creation to take place. Ham kode (empty space) was created.

What does the removal of the infinite light actually mean? Does it mean that Ein Sof actually physically removed the light? A better description would be that Ein Sof hid the light within, throughout, and beyond creation as dark energy, dark matter, atomic matter and the four forces. With the act of tzimtzum, Ein Sof drew back the infinite to create a space in which the finite could be realized.

In Kabbalah an important aspect of this finite light is described as the kav, a single ray of the infinite of Ein Sof and in KST the ohrim, as it descends into creation. Think of this single ray of kav as a single ray of the sun. To gaze into the entirety of the sun's light would be blinding. But by focusing on a single ray, we can appreciate its infinite beauty.

It is only our limited human consciousness that prevents us from seeing Ein Sof in everything and beyond. Thus, the contraction of the light of Ein Sof was and is only from our perspective. From the perspective of Ein Sof, the light continues to be infinite.

Science makes this clear as well. Einstein's famous equation $e=mc2$ describes how light and physical matter are the same substance functioning at different frequencies. Likewise, the kav manifests at different frequencies as would complement the olamot world it is located in. Yet, they are still made of the same material. With discoveries such as the Higgs boson at Cern on 7.4.12, and the quantum robin, this concept became even more tangible to our consciousness. However, even these concepts and discoveries are but a single ray of light within an infinite brilliant sun.

Why then talk about tzimtzum as a contraction? This is for our benefit, to gauge an understanding of the infinite while still allowing us freedom of choice. This is the primary purpose of creation. If we were fully conscious of Ein Sof, there would be no choice; we would only want to act in accordance with the light. Choice is our responsibility and revealing the hidden aspects of the kav via the ohrim into the world and the olamot worlds in a tangible, conscious and healing way is our purpose as KST practitioners.

The act of tzimtzum created something from nothing. The verb bara, used in the first verse of Genesis, expresses this idea. Even prior to tohu (chaos), there was no time or space, so the phrase "in the beginning" had no defined meaning. The letter Bet that is interpreted as "in" can also be interpreted as "with." The Zohar often uses Bet as "with" to imply that space was created "with the beginning." That would make it even easier to see that it was only as the contraction began that time and space created a beginning. However, it is important to consider that the beginning, middle and end of creation already existed and continues to exist within Ein Sof. Creating with the beginning implies the totality of creation existing within Ein Sof prior to creation and being a part of the initial creative process.

So how are we allowed free will if everything has already occurred? This apparent paradox is only due to our limited consciousness. Special Relativity gives us an understanding of times relative nature. Likewise, Chochmah flows in all directions of time and space while tethered to an infinite point. From the perspective of Ein Sof there is room for both pre-determination and free will. Ein Sof can reside fully in the smallest blade of grass as well as any and every point in the olamot worlds simultaneously. It is beyond any restriction that a limited perspective might impose.

As explained by the modern physics of quantum mechanics and quantum biology, their can be a superposition of several different possibilities that simultaneously exist. These reduce to a single possibility after being seen by an observer. By the choices we make, we are participating in our own reality, which is simultaneously enclosed in the infinite perspective and possibility of Ein Sof.

Recall that the kav is the finite version of the infinite light of Ein Sof, likened to a single ray of the sun's light. As the kav descended into creation and/or attenuated within each of the five levels known as the olamot worlds it became the five Sephirotic Trees of Life, one for each olamot world. Each ToL gives substance and definition via particular frequencies of vibration to these primary levels of creation. Within each ToL exists the ten sephirot, the building blocks of all that we know.

This could be likened to the refraction of light through a prism. A single ray produces a variety of magnificent color. In the case of the olamot worlds, the attenuation of the kav as the ToL (and refraction within ZA or Zeir Anpin) results in each level displaying varying qualities of souls, angels, elements and constellations.

All that is called in My Name, for My Glory (Atzilut), I have created it (Beriah), I have formed it (Yetzirah), and I have made it (Asiyah). [27]
— Isaiah (43:7)

This macrocosmic light attenuating into and expressing in various levels of the microcosm is the blueprint for our energy anatomy. These include the Body of Asiyah, Body of Yetzirah, Body of Beriah, Body of Atzilut and Body of Adom Kadmon. They are not separate from their source, but they appear so from our limited human consciousness.

There exist countless levels within these five olamot worlds. We will focus on the five as generalizations. Beginning with the lowest realm, they are referred to as Asiyah, Yetzirah, Beriah, Atzilut and Adam Kadmon.

The fifth level of Adam Kadmon is often not counted in discussions about the olamot worlds. This is due to its nature that mediates between Ein Sof as manifestation beyond time and space and the four lower worlds. It is so far from our ability to comprehend that any attempt to describe it will be less than lacking. However, it plays an important role in the interplay of our physical body with the creation around us and plays a primary role in aspects of healing. Thus, it will continue to be included in the explorations of KSTechnique.

Olamot Worlds and Energy Bodies

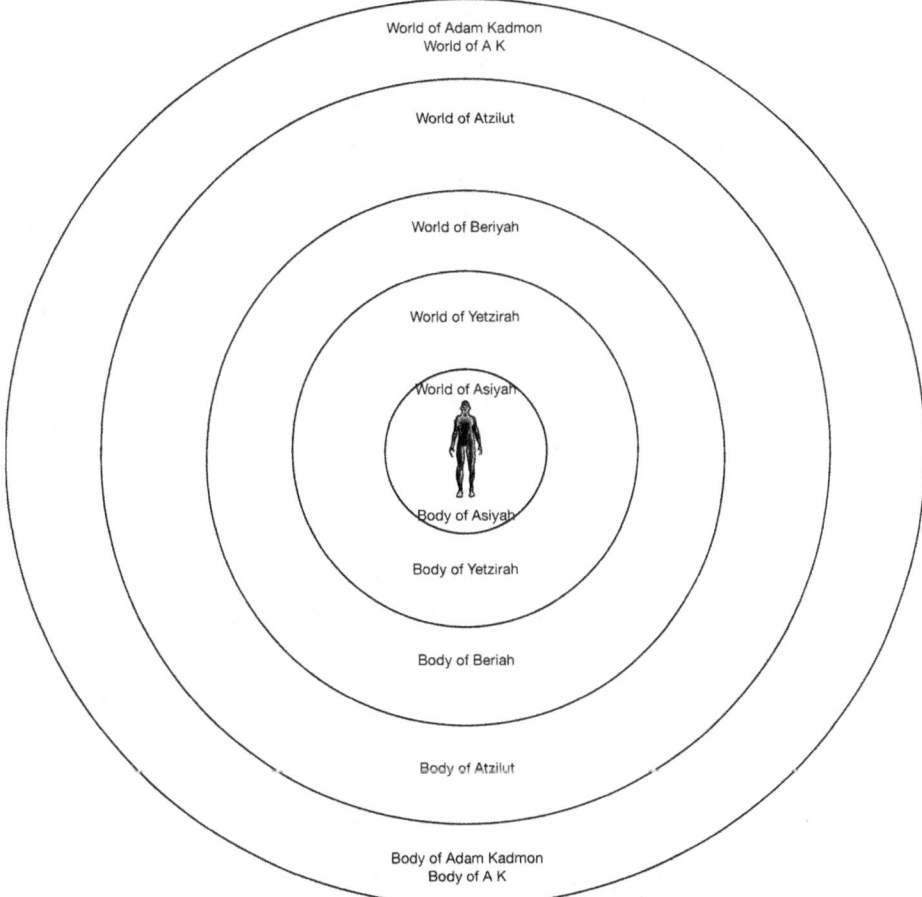

BODY OF ASIYAH

This is described as the effect of the ultimate cause where free will reigns.

Asiyah means making. It is the ultimate effect of the primordial desire to have free will within creation. It is the only olamot world where free will can fully exist. This is because it is the only place where both good and evil can exist in close proximity, thus availing us to the challenges of having choice.

As the frequency of the kav attenuates through Yetzirah, it slows until it becomes the World of Asiyah where it connects with our avir (aura) and becomes the Body of Asiyah, Zelum Elohim and the physical body.

The Zelum Elohim does not have its own section in this chapter because it is inextricably connected to the Body of Asiyah. It may be palpated from the skin to an inch off the body. It is a blueprint of the physical body. This field has been documented in kirlian photography. Some of the first photos taken of Zelum Elohim using this technique were of energy remnants of a leaf. It is called the phantom leaf. The energy form of a leaf can still be photographed via this method even after the leaf has been clipped from its branch and is no longer physically there.

Zelum Elohim is the blueprint for the physical body the same way the Body of Asiyah contains the blueprint for the entire universe. The Body of Asiyah is a reflective vessel for creation. It is the place where time, space and earthly consciousness become a tangible reality.

The angelic forms here are referred to as *ophanim*, meaning wheels. These wheels, as forces, may be likened to the energy centers of our physical bodies. The ophanim extend into all of the energy bodies of our avir. We palpate them with the pendulum during a sephirot reading.

Other angels also coordinate with our physical body. Archangels such as Michael, Gabriel, Uriel, and Raphael have, at times, been made into anthropomorphic representations for us to better relate to personally. However, they are forces far more complex than their human-like counterparts. The archangels, and how they relate to the Body of

Asiyah, will be explored a bit more in chapter fourteen, "Angels." In short, Michael relates to the right side of the body, Gabriel to the left, Uriel to the front and Raphael to the back and/or spine.

BODY OF YETZIRAH

YETZIRAH IS THE WORLD OF FORMATION. It is the realm of emotion. Here, time and space take form, the colors of the rainbow become distinct and duality becomes reality. Yetzirah also is home for the world of angels and/or chayot hakodesh meaning holy animals.

As the frequency of the kav attenuates through the World of Beriah, it slows yet again until it becomes the World of Yetzirah where it connects with our avir (aura) and becomes the Body of Yetzirah. This is our emotional body.

The Body of Yetzirah begins a few inches from the physical body and extends between one to three feet. This is the energy body that we palpate during a KSTechnique® pendulum reading. It is called the emotional body, for it is here that we experience most of our emotions. Emotions, like our thoughts, are differentiated by their various rates of vibration. They reside in their specified olamot world and body according to which frequencies they are in harmony with.

Tremendous emotional healing takes place when working with the Body of Yetzirah. Tears may flow, laughter can be heard or charged memories may surface. This is often the stuck energy of emotions moving through the body. Emotional energy that is stuck is often due to feelings we did not deal with because it felt too painful to do so at the time of their origin. When these emotions are held in our avir or energy field they create an area or clump of slowed down frequency within the quickened one that is in balance. This makes the energy look blotchy or dark.

Usually we must feel the emotions that we've held onto in order to allow them to move and transform. When our energy quickens it will be free to transmute to what it is destined to be. Once we feel the stuck energy and breathe through it, we will be truly free from the blockage and will have attained the lesson from that experience.

Ruah means breath. By learning how to come into contact with our breath we can facilitate healing. This is explored in greater depth in the section on the RT (Ruah Technique) in chapter three. Teaching our clients to connect with their breath this way can aid in moving energy that is stuck in their Body of Yetzirah. Even a few deep breaths during a session can facilitate the release of a block.

As healers we may feel or witness our client's release of stuck emotions. We must allow this experience to move through us and not hold unto it. This can be difficult if our client's emotional trauma mirrors one of our own. Thus, it is of the utmost importance to receive our own healing to resolve personal issues. If our client's issues do stick to us, see it as an opportunity to heal something within that was not previously resolved. Seek professional assistance when needed.

We can only take our clients as far as we have gone ourselves. It is imperative to become as self-aware as possible. This will help to avoid potential pitfalls while doing our work. The more we grow the more we evolve as healers.

A valuable technique prior to a session is to perform RT and remember to hold kavana and not attach to our client's injuries even when they mirror our own. Ask for guidance. This is our client's time and we are there to honor their process. Taking on their injuries makes the session about us and takes away from the client.

BODY OF BERIAH

THE BODY OF BERIAH (mind) contains the consciousness of "I," which allows us to experience ourselves as separate from another in order to have an individual experience of life.

Beriah means distinct creation. It is the first level (above to below) where we begin to discern the concept of our individuality. It is the universal mind. It continues to be highly spiritual in nature, although it is dominated by the innate nature of mind.

The level of Beriah connects with our avir as the Body of Beriah. It is our mental body. Its frequency is slower or attenuated from that of the Body of Atzilut. The Body of Beriah extends outward from the physical body an average of a yard to a yard and a half. The Body of Beriah is associated with the brain in the physical body.

Having a balanced Body of Beriah results in spiritual knowledge and discernment, i.e., clarity of mind. It is golden in color and often in the shape of an egg around the physical body or Body of Asiyah. An imbalanced state may result in narrow linear thinking. It is not the ignorance of innocence, but rather the ignorance of prejudice. In this state, the typically pristine color when in balance gets blotchy and its shape non-symmetrical.

The Body of Beriah sometimes leads to a fascinating interplay with the other energy bodies of avir. It results in our mind receiving information that has been influenced by our physical experience and emotions.

For instance, when the physical senses gather information about the world, this gets pressed through previous life experiences. Then, the information is filtered through the emotional Body of Yetzirah before it gets to our Body of Beriah where the mind processes the filtered information and decides on what we think about the physical event. Sometimes this leads to a decision of how to respond to the event before it has time to reach the spiritual body. The mind in the Body of Beriah sends the message to the physical body through the same emotional Body of Yetzirah on the way to delivering that information to the physical Body of Asiyah. The physical senses filter through an unresolved emotional charge felt in the emotional Body of Yetzirah. The result is often misinterpretation and bias. Thus, for mental clarity in life it is imperative to provide assistance for clearing and harmonizing the Body of Yetzirah (emotions) and the other bodies.

One way to help clear our energetic anatomy is to seek our information from the Body of Atzilut and integrate this information into the bodies at the levels of Beriah, Yetzirah and Asiyah (in that sequence) in order to bring harmony with universal law. Doing this same clearing process, via beginning with the lower frequencies in the physical Body of Asiyah, will work as well but can take lifetimes!

BODY OF ATZILUT

The Sephirot of Nothingness...

—*Sefer Yetzirah,* Ayreh Kaplan

ATZILUT MAINTAINS THE NEXT HIGHEST LEVEL of spiritual vibration next to that of Adam Kadmon. In Atzilut time and space are still not fully manifest, yet the potential of manifestation is more fully formed. It is where past, present and future intermingle. Linear time breaks down. Accessing information and records of the past, future or present may be done here.

It is called the level of nothingness or ein in Hebrew. Atzilut is virtually indistinguishable from the universal healing light or ohrim that we become vessels for during healing sessions.

The sephirot become distinguishable here and Atzilut is considered their domain. Since this is a level of nothingness, the sephirot on this level are referred to as the "Sephirot of Nothingness"[29] in the Sefer Yetzirah, one of the primary ancient texts of Kabbalah.

The realm of Atzilut connects to our avir as the Body of Atzilut. This is our causal body. The Body of Atzilut energetically extends outward from the physical body an average of a few yards. In the case of a spiritually evolved being, this energy body may reach out as far as a mile.

Through this magnificent, transcendent energy field, we can experience unity with all creation while still maintaining a semblance of our individual potential. If our consciousness becomes attune to this vibration we begin to gain insight into our life's true purpose. We see the bigger picture of our life.

The Body of Atzilut, along with the Body of Adam Kadmon, is said to transcend the physical anatomy of the Body of Asiyah. These are the two levels where we would attempt to place our neutral kavana or intention when facilitating the flow of ohrim during distance healing.

Both the level of Adam Kadmon and the level of Atzilut are excellent for distance healing. The primary difference is that our kavana is best placed on Adam Kadmon during general sessions, whereas the kavana should be focused on Atzilut during sessions that are specific to linear time.

For example, sessions that involve time and space bound issues it is best to focus your kavana on the level of Atzilut where time and space have form albeit non-linear. For instance, if a client wants closure for a past relationship, the level of Atzilut would be good to focus on.

BODY OF ADAM KADMON

... ascending in thought, in inner mystery (Hebrew) (Et ha-adam), human-mystery of male and female as one. [28]
—*Zohar*, Daniel C. Matt

THE BODY OF ADAM KADMON touches the true reality that encompasses all of creation and its purpose. Although this level is beyond human comprehension, it is still a creation and, from our perspective, separate from Ein Sof or infinity.

Adam Kadmon is the highest level of creation and is the closest to the frequency of Ein Sof. It is closest to the divine source in a linear sense. Our avir, or energy field, on this level is called the Body of Adam Kadmon. This body is our spiritual body. It is the potential of all form including our own human form. It is the potential of primordial human. Its energy extends indefinitely.

Here the potential for all creation exists. Even time and space exist only as potential. Every potential of form and formlessness exist simultaneously both with and without time and with and without space. It is mate-ve-lo-mate as creation. It is like the primordial light before it cooled and became the four forces of nature.

In our esoteric anatomy the Body of Adam Kadmon is likened to the web of life. It extends beyond our individual energy field of avir to connect us with all of creation and beyond. To be in touch with it is to have a unification experience. This is the power of our interconnection with the universe beyond our sense of individuality and beyond our concept of time and space.

Chapter 12

Healing Symbols

Whoever bears that sign passes through all gates above, with no one hindering him. [30]

—*Zohar,* Daniel C. Matt

HEBREW LETTERS HAVE BEEN UTILIZED as an ancient and modern writing tool for thousands of years. As an ancient language, the letters found their expression in many sacred texts. The letters were written down physically, yet they are much more than script. In esoteric texts, such as the Sefer Yetzirah and other teachings of Kabbalah, we find that these same letters become symbols which hold a much deeper energy. These symbols have the ability to teach us lessons related to us, our world and to healing.

In addition to their function as script, the form and sound of the individual Hebrew letters have an energetic and symbolic meaning with tangible and appreciable effects when used correctly. When viewing the meaning from this deeper perspective, these letters exist as energetic forces. Sometimes these forces act as symbols that are a filter for the universal healing light of ohrim.

Hebrew letters do not change what they are in order to become healing symbols. Rather it is our consciousness that shifts in order to see the broader capacity they contain. Even that is but a fraction of the energy contained within them. However, considering the limited capacity of human beings to embrace the ohrim (universal healing light), this is plenty! The previous statement is not to demean humanity, rather it is intended to recognize how we are created and honor it by working within our human limitations.

Our limits are what give us free will, which is one of our greatest gifts. Using free will to choose to become a source for healing is a perfect way to honor that gift and begin to fulfill our potential.

As symbols, the letters help us learn and explore all that we have studied in KST. It is another component for healing. By exploring the sephirot and olamot worlds via the symbols, we are exploring the corresponding areas of ourselves and others that we are guided to help heal.

Letters have a distinct character that allows them to act as tools for healing. They refract the ohrim in ways that facilitate healing intent. It is our responsibility as healers to develop our abilities as much as possible in order to fulfill our intention to heal even though the wisdom of the ohrim knows where to go. This is an aspect of free will that may seem contradictory, but it is not. Developing our consciousness as healers mirrors the ohrim. To integrate that understanding results in a profound experience that honors free will.

The symbols help guide us on our path. All that is required is our ability to hear their expression correctly. When we avail ourselves to the direction of the ohrim with a pure and willing heart our experiences will be the correct ones for us.

TETRAGRAMMATON AS A TOOL FOR HEALING

THE TETRAGRAMMATON IS ONE of the most powerful healing combinations of Hebrew letters we have. It is made up of three letters: Yud, Hey and Vav. The Hey is used twice making it Yud, Hey, Vav and Hey.

We visualize the tetragrammaton in our mind's eye during meditation. Imagine the letters as black fire on white fire. Our mind is at

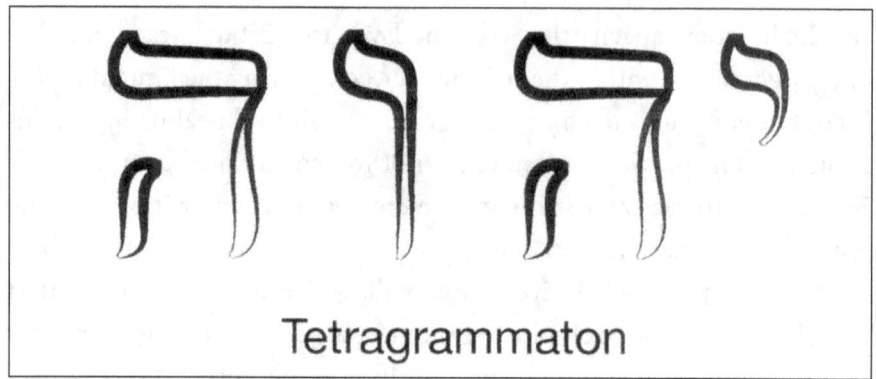

Tetragrammaton

rest while we visualize. Do not attempt to control random thoughts that may intrude. See these thoughts as clouds in a blue sky and simply allow them to float by. Then, refocus on the tetragrammaton.

Each letter-symbol of the tetragrammaton corresponds to a different level of creation (olamot world), energy body, and sephirah. Knowing which symbol is linked to which of these levels let's us know what type of healing the symbol is ideal for. For instance, since the body of the letter Yud refers to the Sephirah of Chochmah, the spiritual Body of Atzilut in the World of Atzilut, we know that this letter would be appropriate for use in spiritual healing.

Attunements

Becoming attuned to a letter as a symbol means becoming aware of its meaning on a deeper level. The letter becomes a visual symbol of a larger spiritual concept. We activate our awareness and direct the symbols energy during healing sessions. The more we practice, the easier the ohrim (universal healing light) flows.

To 'activate' a letter means to turn it on, to make it work or go into action.

In order to activate and work with the symbols as a healing tool, we must attune to them. In KSTechnique® this is ideally done via an attunement session with a KSM teacher. A series of simple exercises will help you to connect to the symbols you will be working with on an ongoing basis. These exercises assist in forming a personal relationship

Healing Symbols

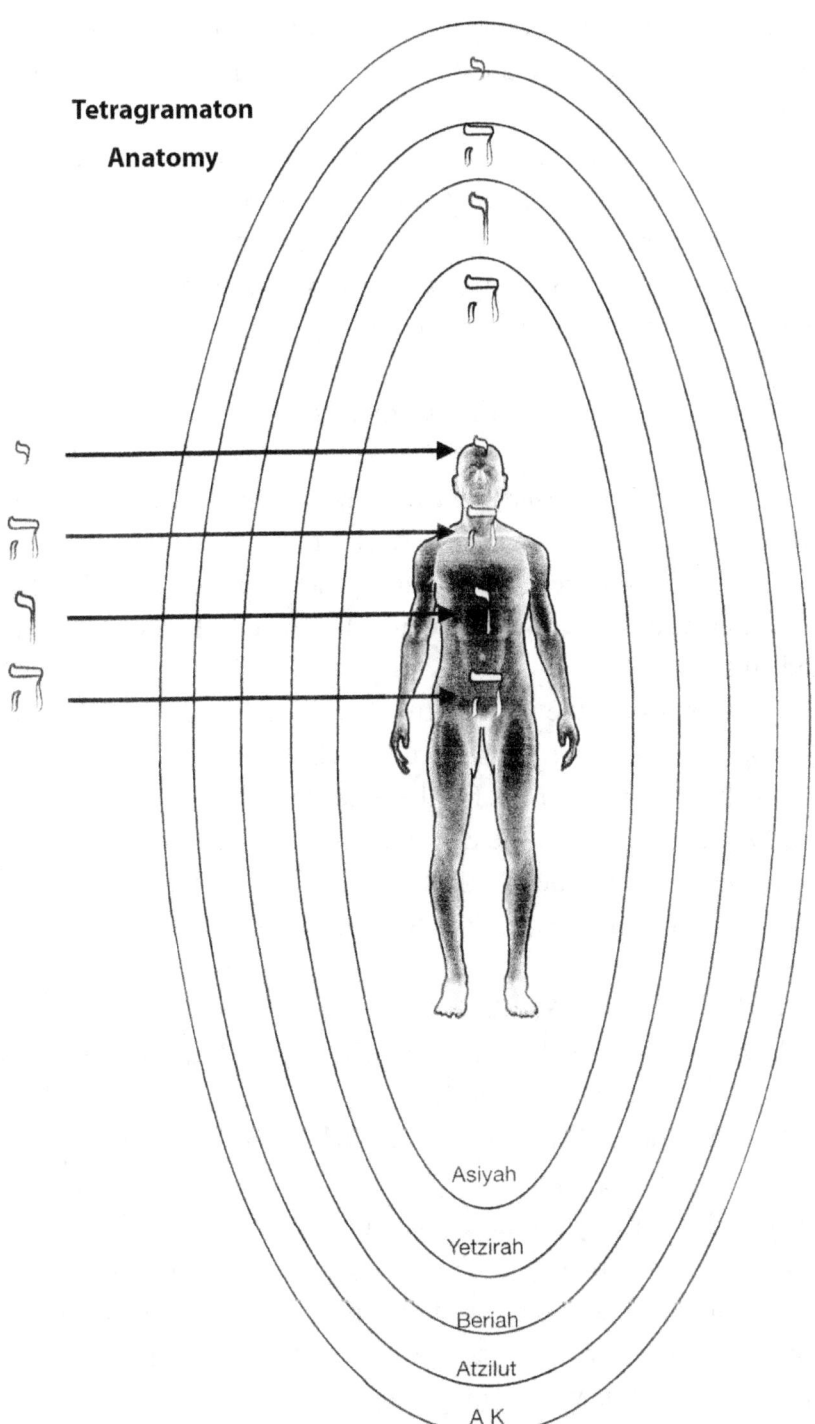

with the symbols. We develop a deeper awareness of their meaning. In KSP II classes we explore the three letters Yud, Hey and Vav as healing symbols.

The ability to utilize the letters as healing tools can still be accomplished without an attunement session, however, it is highly recommended in order to receive a direct transmission of the energy. There are several ways to activate the letters once you have been attuned to them. Some examples are described below:

Symbol Connections

The symbol for the lower letter of Hey is related to the World and Body of Asiyah and the Sephirot of Malchut.

The symbol for the letter of Vav is related to the World and Body of Yetzirah and the Sephirot of Chesed, Gevurah, Tipheret, Netzach, Hod and Yesod.

The symbol for the upper letter Hey is related to the World and Body of Beriah and the Sephirah of Binah.

The body of the symbol for the letter Yud is related to the World and Body of Atzilut and the Sephirah of Chochmah.

The tip of the symbol for the letter Yud is related to the World and Body of Adom Kadmon and the Sephirah of Keter.

Activating Letters as Symbols

Ideally a healer will have an attunement session with an already initiated KSM practitioner. This allows the energy of the symbol to flow directly where it is needed with ease. The KST practitioner will find their practice intensified. Only a person who has been attuned as a teacher level practitioner may attune a healer in this manner.

Activate a symbol by thinking, visualizing or feeling its name, by speaking it out loud or silently or drawing it either internally or externally. The more attuned we become to the letters as symbols of a deeper truth, the easier this will become.

"Drawing" a letter as a symbol in KSTechnique® is a multi-layered reference. It can mean to physically draw the symbol on paper or on a photo of the intended recipient, to trace the letter in the air with our finger or visualize drawing them in our mind. The method used to draw the symbol does not make a difference and may vary with circumstances. For example, if we are with a group of people and need to draw the Lower Hey for protection it might be a challenge to physically draw the letter in the air. For reasons of privacy we could simply visualize drawing it in front and around ourselves. It is good to be versatile.

The following few pages have a breakdown of how to utilize each of the four letters of the tetragrammaton as a healing tool.

LOWER HEY

Power symbol

OUR PHYSICAL WORLD of Asiyah is only ten percent of what exists in creation. And of that ten percent, we are only conscious of a small percentage. The Lower Hey helps to bring the ohrim from the other ninety percent of the energetic realms to a specified physical location. If at any time you desire to increase the magnification of the ohrim that you are offering, activate this letter.

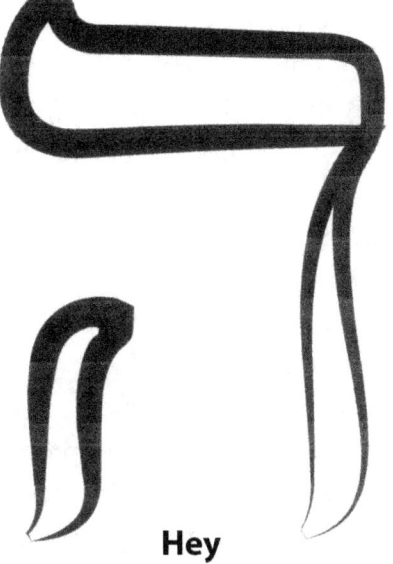
Hey

As you recall, the upper level of Hey is associated with mental healing. The Lower Hey is perfect for protection and physical healing. This symbol helps to increase the power of ohrim to the area directed and needed. Whether being used for healing or protection, this symbol magnifies the ohrim. By activating the Lower Hey you are saying, "place the ohrim of Ein Sof here."

If at any time during a session you want to increase the power of ohrim, all you have to do is activate this symbol. The Lower Hey can also be directed to focus ohrim on a specific location, person or intention. It may be utilized at any time. For instance, we may choose to begin a session with this symbol to intensify the strength of the session. Then we may use it to seal in healing at the completion of the session. Any increase of ohrim will help facilitate the elevation of sparks in a client's tikkun process.

The Lower Hey may also be used for protection. Draw the Lower Hey around or within the area we want to protect. This technique can be utilized for us, our client, house, kids, cat, car, birds, Earth, universe, tree or anything or anyone we feel requires protection. For instance, we may wish to draw the Lower Hey around a car before we get into it or around a plane prior to a flight.

The Lower Hey is associated with the Body of Asiyah. It is connected with the Sephirah of Malchut, which is the 'effect' of the 'cause' of creation. This symbol says, 'place the ohrim of Ein Sof here.'

Use it for protection and physical healing.

Exercises:
1. Draw the Lower Hey on a blank piece of paper 108 times.
2. Perform RT (Ruah Technique) with the Hey imagined at your pelvis or feet.
3. Draw the Hey in the air in each corner of the room or in the center of the room for protection.
4. If a partner is available, pair up. Activate the Lower Hey and perform a short version of the sephirot assessment and protocol.

VAV

Emotional Healer

VAV IS THE SYMBOL FOR EMOTIONAL HEALING. It is perfect for aiding the healing process of personal trauma and blocks. Vav resides in the Body of Yetzirah, the emotional body. The Vav is a truly wonderful symbol for getting to the heart of what ails us.

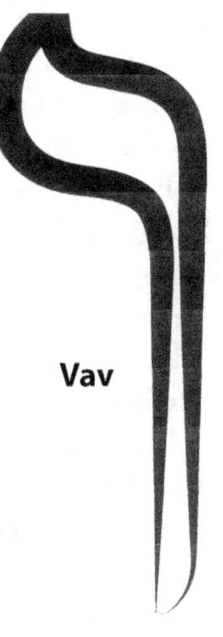

Vav

Our emotions are directly affected by our mind and our body. This is due to the emotions placement in our esoteric anatomy. The emotional Body of Yetzirah resides above our physical Body of Asiyah (Lower Hey) and below our mental Body of Beriah (Upper Hey).

When the Vav and Hey are used during a treatment session there is a synergistic effect. Emotional issues can be approached through the mind during counseling sessions since the mind is linked to the emotions from above. Emotional issues can be approached through the body during bodywork sessions since the body is linked to the emotions from below. Both therapies require training. Both therapies can use the Hey and Vav together for a synergistic effect. When counseling and bodywork are combined the effect is magnified ten-fold. In many jurisdictions the counselor and the bodyworker are different individuals requiring different licenses. They can work together as a treatment team.

Use these symbols when working with relationship issues, depression, nervous disorders, fear, anger or the like. The Vav is like energetic psychotherapy. The other symbols help guide our emotional healing process but it is Vav that accomplishes it. For instance, we can mentally identify how an emotional block came to be yet still be triggered by it. Knowing how an issue came to be is helpful in directing us to what needs to be healed and why but that is not enough. By utilizing Vav we feel the injury and move its energy through the Body of Yetzirah. We know the emotional injury has healed when we are no longer triggered by it.

Our emotions drive our desires and actions. This is not always a conscious process. Most of our actions are subconsciously motivated and much of that motivation stems from emotional issues. To uncover, help heal and be released from these issues is to become conscious of our motivations and intentions.

Bringing our subconscious awareness into consciousness is helped through mythology that mirrors the truth of our existence. It is the language of our emotions. In Kabbalah this language exactly describes the healing aspect of Vav. It says that by releasing our emotional issues we help to elevate sparks (enlightened parts of us and the universe) that are trapped within our emotional wounding.

The term "sparks" refers to sparks of the original light ray of Ein Sof called the kav. During creation, this light poured forth through the eyes of Adam Kadmon (primordial form) and was gathered and held at the level of Atzilut within the primitive ten vessels of the sephirot. These vessels were not capable of holding the divine light and therefore, at the level of Malchut, the vessels shattered. Some of the light scattered and became sparks. These sparks failed to return to the primordial source. Instead, they became attached and trapped in the broken fragments of the vessels, causing the divine light of creation to "fall into matter." This is another way of describing the primordial light of the Big Bang as it cooled into the four forces and matter.

We are now living in a cosmic stage in which the process of restoration, healing and repair must be undertaken. This process is known as "tikkun." Activating the letter Vav helps to facilitate individual healing as well as the healing of our world as a whole.

As practitioners we must also take care of ourselves. Activate Vav regularly as part of a personal journey towards emotional well-being. This helps us stay emotionally balanced. It's not easy to overcome our traumas or issues. They become our shadow when left hidden. The more we heal ourselves, the more we grow toward our potentials in life.

In our professional practice we can only take a client as far as we have gone. The more we heal ourselves the further we can take our clients and the more we can become stable vessels for helping to heal the world one person at a time.

We activate Vav as a healing symbol at the start of a session. For example: if we are a psychotherapist and our client is sad, the kavana might be to help alleviate the sadness. Or, if we are a bodyworker and are doing an energy hold at the opening of a session on a prone client, we can hold one hand on the sacrum and the other on the foot. When we feel the energy connect, we trace the Vav along the client's spine and foot at the same time. Hold. We release the foot and hold the other foot while continuing the contact on the client's back with our other hand. We hold until we feel the energy connect. Then we trace the Vav on the back and the other foot. Hold. Release. Continue with the session.

The Vav has a numerical value of 6 and coordinates with ZA (Zeir Anpin). The six Sephirot of ZA are called Chesed, Gevurah, Tipheret, Netzach, Hod and Yesod.

Vav is associated with the emotional Body of Yetzirah.

Vav is like energetic psychotherapy.

Exercises:

1. Draw Vav 108 times on a blank sheet of paper.
2. Perform RT and imagine Vav as your torso.
3. Take a photo of yourself or someone who has agreed to receive this emotional healing. Visualize or draw Vav on the photo. Place or hold the photo on your solar plexus until you feel the flow of the ohrim. At the same time, hold healing kavana in your heart.

UPPER HEY

Healer of the Mind

(He)-why is it Binah? He replied, Come and see what is written: A river issues from Eden to water the garden (Genesis 2:10). Who is the river that issues from Eden? Binah. Hence, (he) is the river, and (yod) is enclosed within Her.[32]

— *Zohar,* Daniel C. Matt

THE TETRAGRAMMATON CONTAINS TWO LEVELS of the symbol Hey. The upper Hey is associated with mental healing (using the mind to heal) as well as being a healer of the mind. Hey resides with understanding or the Sephirah of Binah, the Divine Mother who gives birth to the physical world.

Utilizing Hey as a way toward balancing our thoughts is key as we seek to understand the mind and its processes. Incorporating the Upper Hey into a counseling practice will help facilitate the flow of understanding, growth and healing of any imbalance of the mind. Psychologists, psychotherapists and counselors can all benefit from this technique in their practice.

Hey has the numerical value of five which corresponds to the five fingers, five elements, the five senses, and the five dimensions. This is the level where duality begins. Therefore, the Upper Hey is where negativity begins to exist as a dual to positivity. This is also where our free will begins.

This is a truly wonderful symbol for getting to the details of what is troubling our mind. A secondary location for the mind is our heart. This is the secondary placement of the Sephirah of Binah in the body. In KST we call this our heart-mind. It is where our emotions and our mind meet. When in balance, the wisdom of the heart-mind can lead us to clarity, insight and blessing on a feeling level.

Hey is a wonderful tool to use for the alleviations of mental fatigue, mental confusion, addictions, anxiety, memory problems, or unwanted habits. This symbol is often utilized in conjunction with the symbol of Vav, as many ailments, such as addiction have both a strong mental and an emotional component.

When working with a client, we may activate this symbol during a session in response to their need for psychological balance, clarity and healing.

Upper Hey is associated with the mental Body of Beriah. It is also connected to the Sephirot of Binah and the many blessings we have in our life.

Exercises:
1. Draw Hey 108 times on a blank sheet of paper.
2. Perform the RT (Ruah Technique). Then imagine Hey between your brows or in your heart center.
3. Take a photo of yourself or someone who needs mental healing and place it between your hands. Hold kavana for the mental healing of the person in the photo. Feel the ohrim flow. Allow understanding to guide you.

YUD

Healer of the Soul

Within concealment of the concealed was engrained an engraving, invisible, unrevealed. [31]

— *Zohar,* Daniel C. Matt

YUD IS THE HEALER OF THE SOUL. This symbol may be used in every session, especially distance healing. It is a perfect choice for spiritual healing. Since it originates above negativity, it aids us in pulling negativity out of the body and transforming it into loving healing energy. This symbol has the capacity to take our healing abilities to their highest level possible. It expands our awareness and consciousness.

At its origin, all energy is unconditional love. Only at the level of the Sephirah of Binah and below does this original energy begin

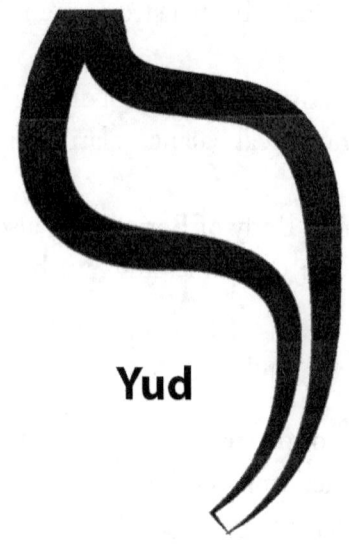

Yud

to express as the duality of positive and negative. This dual state offers us free will and the challenges that come with choices.

When we activate Yud we allow energy to reach beyond the Sephirah of Binah, to the energy's origin of pure and undifferentiated love. At the level of our physical existence, we are not capable of observing the larger picture where the path of true healing is known.

Energy appears to express itself negatively or positively. This dualistic effect helps to continue a lesson, offer a challenge, or perform another service in our life. We must let go of strict judgment and remain neutral in our role as facilitators of healing. We must trust that, if our kavana (intention) is pure, the best possible outcome will occur.

The Yud begins at the crown or Sephirah of Keter in the World of Adom Kadmon. On this level, we only find the tip of the symbol Yud as a small point. Activating this symbol helps us work with the Body of Adom Kadmon, the outermost part of our avir (energy body). The small point is the center of creation. That center is limitless and is found throughout the universe. It creates a weblike connection with everything. This is the perfect symbol to use with any KST distance healing technique. Working with this energy compliments any work being done with the Sephirot of Keter. Any form of distance healing will be magnified through the use of Yud.

The body of the Yud is rooted in wisdom or the Sephirah of Chochmah in the World of Atzilut. Yud is a master symbol. When we activate this symbol during a session it intensifies the spiritual flow of the ohrim in all directions and in all time. The body of Yud is indicated when time and space need to be considered. For instance, if our client is undergoing surgery a week from the session we are in, we can activate the body of the Yud and set our kavana for healing for that time and place.

When combined with other symbols, Yud takes them to their highest potential of effectiveness. We take our session to a higher vibration and create a strong connection with the spiritual realm when we activate Yud.

Yud is associated with the spiritual level of Atzilut. The tip of the Yud is associated with the Sephirot of Keter and the Body of Adam Kadmon. The body of the Yud works with the Sephirah of Chochmah and the Body of Atzilut.

Exercises:
1. Draw Yud 108 times.
2. Perform RT with a dot imagined at the crown of your head or the full Yud between your brows.
3. Visualize or draw the letter in the air and surround yourself in it.
4. Activate the tip of Yud and perform a ToL reading from a distance.
5. Hold a picture of someone who wants healing and imagine the body of Yud surrounding them.

Chapter 13

Three Constitutions, Three Mothers, Three Symbols

Three Mothers AMSh in the Soul, male and female, are the head, belly, and chest. The head is created from fire, The belly is created from water and the chest, from breath decides between them.[33]
— *Sefer Yetzirah*, Aryeh Kaplan

VIEWING THE ToL from a horizontal perspective offers great insight into ourselves and the world around us. It begins with the Three Mothers. The mothers differentiate the ToL into three sections that describe how the five elements of aether, air, fire, water and earth coordinate in our body. This determines our individual constitutions of Air, Fire or Water. Each of these constitutions describe how our body and mind interact with the world.

KSTechnique® approaches the Three Mothers as a person's individual constitution. In KST we assess a client's constitution to help determine their individual treatment needs. This does not change the definition of the Three Mothers. Rather, it makes them accessible to us as a comprehensive healing tool. Once we assess a client's constitution, we can determine which elements are out of balance in the body and recommend ways to bring the client back into balance.

Shin, Aleph and Mem are Hebrew letters. When utilized as symbols they represent the Three Mothers and their associated constitutions.

Three Constitutions

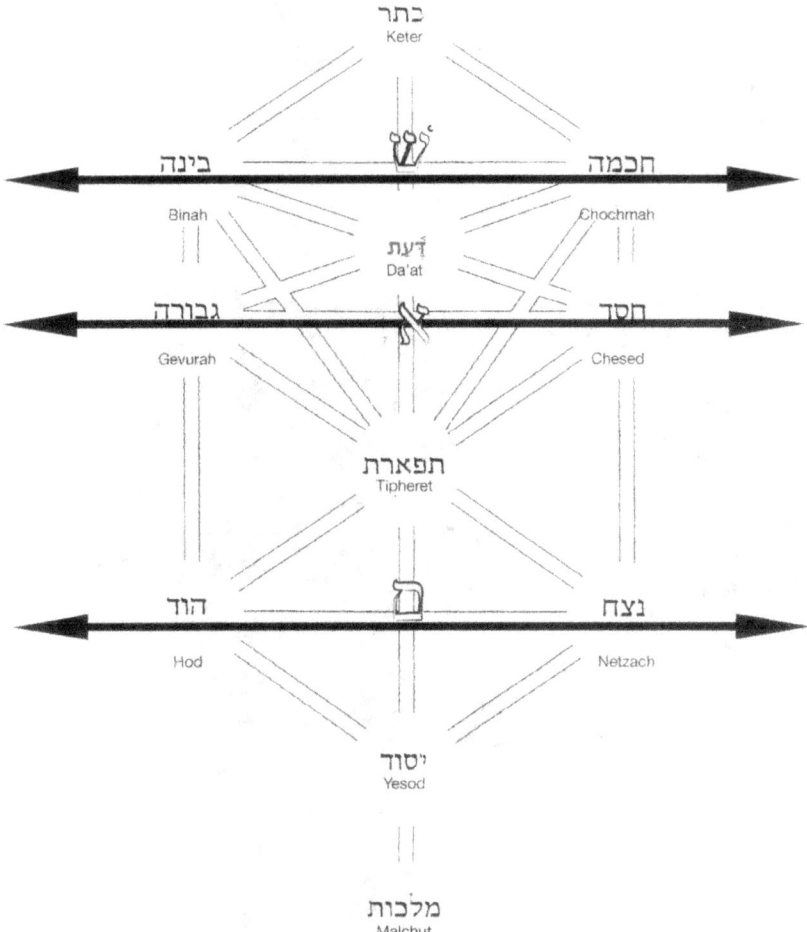

The head is represented by the letter-symbol Shin. The chest is Aleph. The belly is Mem. Each symbol matches a location within the body.

Each symbol and location are then associated with an element. Shin as the head is the element of fire. Aleph as the chest is the element of air. Mem as the belly is the element of water.

Shin is the Fire Constitution. Aleph is the Air Constitution, and Mem is the Water Constitution. A person's constitution can be determined through a pulse test, questionnaire or intake assessment.

Shin
Fire Constitution
Fire Element
Runs Hot
Head
Medium Build
Clear, Leader
Prone to Anger

Aleph
Air Constitution
Aether and Air Elements
Runs Cold
Torso
Slim Build
Open Minded, Creative
Prone to Anxiety

Mem
Water Constitution
Water and Earth Elements
Runs Cool
Pelvis
Heavy Build
Calm, Generous
Prone to Inertia

Elemental Constitutions

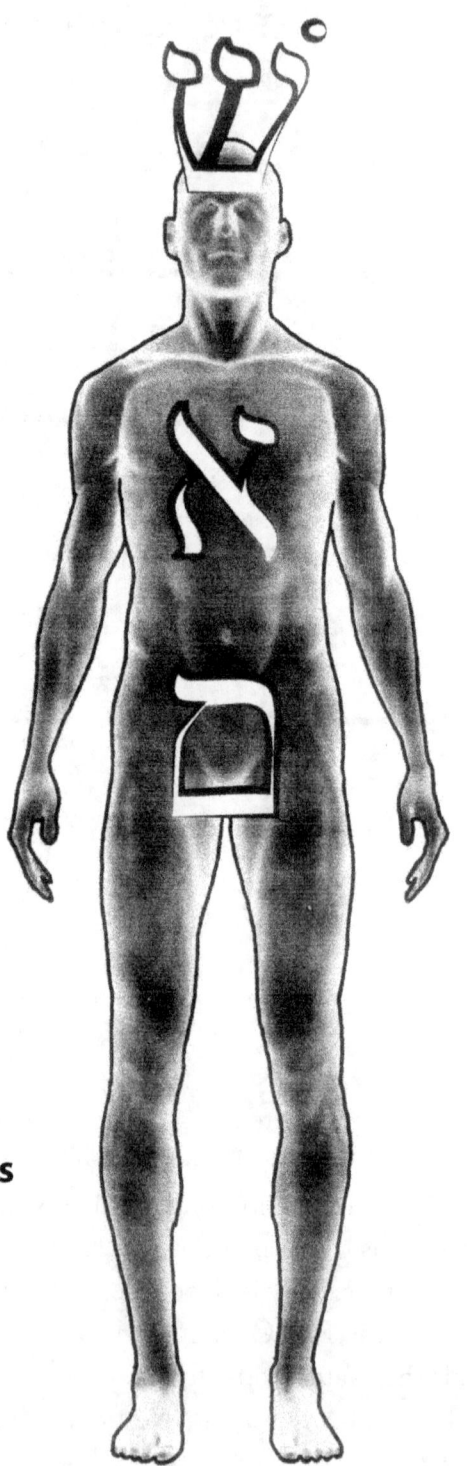

We each have two primary constitutions. They are the underlying constitution we are born with and the presenting constitution that is ever changing depending on environment and circumstances. For instance, if we become cold easily but have recently moved to a low desert during the summer, we may find ourselves overheating. In this case, a typical assessment of an underlying Air Constitution might present as a Fire Constitution and require a KST fire protocol to become balanced during a treatment session. Our underlying Air Constitution has not changed but our presenting imbalance of fire has. Once the presenting imbalance of fire is attended to through cooling, the underlying constitution of Air can be helped by putting a warm sweater back on.

These assessments help us know which of the elements in the body are dominant or out of balance. Then we can remedy the imbalance. In each case, the ToL doesn't change. Rather, it is our perception that shifts depending on our vantage point.

In the treatment setting, a constitutional assessment can be done prior to the reading of the sephirot. This gives depth to a session. Combining the two formats is synergistic. The results give a multifaceted view of the ToL within the body. This is ideal when a client's presenting issue is complex or not overtly obvious. The paragraphs that follow show the connection between the three constitutions and the sephirot.

Individual constitutions and their sephirotic associations are:

1. Fire Constitution relates to the fire element, is located at the head and is represented by the symbol of Shin. It resides on the line between the Sephirot of Chochmah and Binah.
2. Air Consitution relates to the air element, is located at the chest and is represented by the symbol of Aleph. It resides on the line between the Sephirot of Chesed and Gevurah.
3. Water Consitution relates to the water element, is located at the belly and is represented by the symbol of Mem. It resides on the line between the Sephirot of Netzach and Hod as seen from the back of the body.

Three Pillars

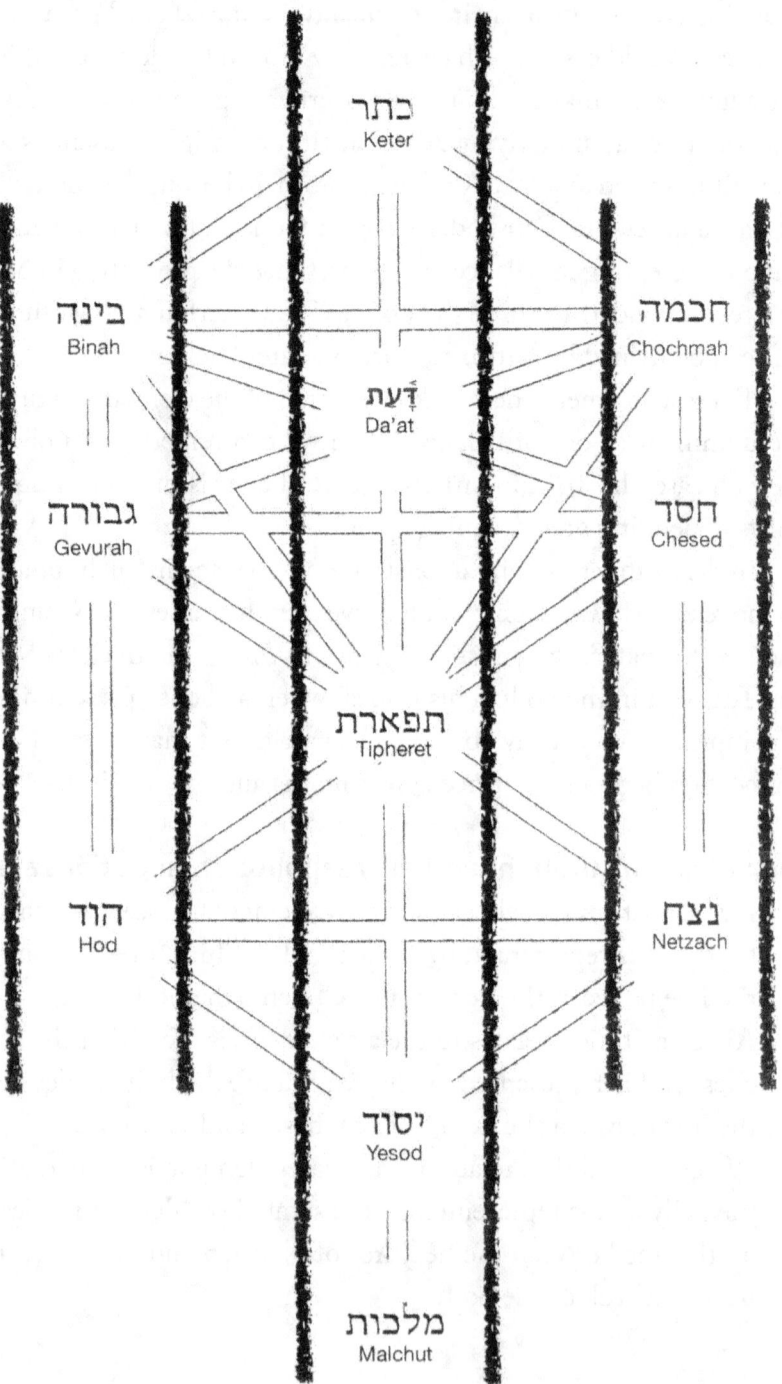

Keeping these three constitutions in balance is vitally important for optimal health and well-being. The three constitutions describe how the five elements coordinate in the body. Aether and air combine to make the Air Constitution. Fire and Water combine to make the Fire Constitution. Water and earth combine to make the Water Constitution. Water is a part of two constitutions. This mirrors our physical body, which is composed of two-thirds water as it overflows into two of the constitutions. It also reflects our connection to the earth, which is covered in two-thirds water.

There are a variety of tools that can aid in maintaining balance with the constitutions. They include bodywork protocols, essential oils, crystals, diet, exercise, meditation, correct diet, psychotherapy, etc.

During the assessment phase of treatment sessions, we establish which of the elements is dominant within a person's body (various techniques to help in this process are given later in this section). We use these same techniques when doing an assessment on ourselves. By determining our presenting constitution or which constitution and element is dominant in the moment, we can help to determine what primary characteristics, lifestyle, dietary, psychological and bodywork adjustments might be helpful. In doing so, we can aid in bringing ourselves more into balance.

Self-care is important when working with others. Maintaining balance is imperative if we are to be conduits of healing for others. This is because when we are sick, all of our energy is spent on regaining health. By maximizing our personal health, we are able to spend more time and energy on areas that facilitate our growth as healers. By keeping ourselves in balance, we are in a position to help bring balance and healing to the world.

THREE CONSTITUTIONS

Fire Constitution

Fire Constitution is related to the Sephirah of Binah and the left side of the ToL. It is regarded as the seat of understanding and articulate thought. The fiery nature of this constitution makes for a driven, intense and extroverted personality. Fire fuels passion, directs intention and transforms us. It sets the boundaries where we define our life.

Fire Constitution embodies the elements of fire and water. It is hot, moist and active. When Fire Constitution is in balance there is a feeling of fairness, justice and centered ambition. The mind is sharp and intelligent. When out of balance, Fire is quick to anger, judgment and frustration.

To help maintain balance, individuals with Fire Constitution need to:
- Stay cool, eat mild foods and breathe through anger.
- Some helpful essential oils are sandalwood, jasmine and lemon.
- Gems include: citrine, sunstone, ruby and tiger's eye.
- Foods should be mild and cool.
- Although this body type tends to crave spices and caffeine, it is best to avoid these during times of imbalance.
- Eating a few balanced meals per day is recommended.
- These constitutions are usually of medium build and weight.
- Exercise such as yoga, weights or swimming is ideal.

Fire relates to the head when viewed from the horizontal perspective of the ToL It is associated with the left column of the ToL when assessing the body from the vertical perspective.

Air Constitution

Air Constitution is associated with the Sephirah of Keter. Once Aether is touched by creation it becomes accessible to us as air in the central column of the ToL. The airy nature of this constitution makes for a creative, open minded and flexible personality. It is the part of our consciousness that is the observer. Air is consciousness of thought and the act of breathing. Air coordinates with the breath and thus *decides between* the constitution of Fire and Water. In doing so, Air has trace qualities of both Fire and Water, in addition to its own airy nature. Air is both conscious and unconscious. We breathe with unconscious intent, as we do during sleep or conscious intent during RT (Ruah Technique). The greater control we gain over our breath the more conscious we become in our life.

Air Constitution reflects the elements of air and aether. It is quick, changeable, wise and creative. When Air Constitution is in balance, a feeling of energetic enthusiasm, insight and creative vitality are at play while the mind remains calm, active, clear and alert. When out of balance, Air is erratic, anxious and nervous.

To help maintain balance, individuals with Air Constitution need to:
- Stay warm, have a regular routine and remain calm.
- Some helpful essential oils are: rose, frankincense and white lotus.
- Gems include: diamond, clear quartz, amethyst and labradorite.
- Foods should be cooked, bland and warm. This is the only constitution that requires red meat, although all may partake when in balance.
- Air Constitution is generally on the slimmer side, at times finding it difficult to gain weight. It is recommended people with this constitution eat a small amount every couple of hours in order to maintain both weight and a

consistent energy level. When there is excessive weight gain the fatty areas are usually smooth, like an inflated balloon.
- Exercise such as yoga is ideal.

Air Constitution relates to the thoracic or lung area when considering the body from the horizontal view of the ToL (Tree of Life). It is associated with the central column of the ToL when assessing the body from the vertical perspective.

Water Constitution

Water Constitution relates to the Sephirah of Chochmah and the right column of the ToL. It is the source of our wisdom and abstract thought. The watery nature of this constitution makes for a deeply emotional, thoughtful and fluid personality. It encompasses our subconscious world. When chochmah consciousness descends into our body as ZA (Zeir Anpin) it becomes the love of giving and unconscious flow of the right column. We connect with our bliss in the world. It is located around the pelvis and under the navel. For this reason many mystics contemplate their belly when attempting to attain chochmah consciousness.

Water Constitution reflects the element of water and earth. It is moist and cool. When the symbol of Mem as the Water Constitution is in balance there is a generous and friendly feeling which may express itself as loving kindness, while the mind is calm and fluid. When Water Constitution is out of balance, a stuck or lazy feeling may take hold.

To help maintain balance, individuals with Water Constitution need to:
- Keep warm, change up their routines from time to time and stay motivated.
- Some helpful essential oils are: orange, peppermint and eucalyptus.
- Gems include: ruby, garnet, hematite and smokey quartz.

Three Constitutions, Three Mothers, Three Symbols

- Foods are best eaten raw and warm. Lighter foods and very little meat are optimal. Eating heavier in the morning and lighter in the evening may be helpful.
- Water types tend to be on the heavy side, at times finding it difficult to lose excess weight.
- Rigorous exercise such as weight lifting, running and aerobics is ideal.

Water Constitution relates to the belly or pelvic area. This can be seen from the horizontal view of the ToL (Tree of Life). It is associated with the right column of the ToL when assessing the body from the vertical perspective.

Attributes of the Three Constitutions

Fire Constitution:
Critical of self and others
Don't like cold foods or drinks
Don't like hot weather
Easily irritable
Efficient
Feel hot often
Impatient
Need regular meals
Organized and accurate
Strong willed
Sweat easily

Air Constitution:
Anxious
Difficulty focusing
Don't gain weight easily
Don't like cold weather
Dry skin

Emotional by nature
Energy in bursts
Indecisive
Irregular sleeper and eater
Lively and enthusiastic
Quick, active
Quick learner, quick forgetter

Water Constitution:
Affectionate, forgiving and peaceful
Calm and composed
Don't anger easily
Gain weight easily
Need eight hours of sleep
Prone to Inertia
Sensitive to cold and damp weather
Skip meals easily
Slow learner but good memory
Slow, methodical and relaxed
Sound sleeper
Steady energy level
Tend to have congestion problems

Written Constitutional Assessment

Please circle which letter best describes you. For instance, if your skeletal structure is slight, circle A. If your skeletal structure is moderate, circle B and if it is large, circle C.

Skeletal Structure:
A) Slight bone structure
B) Moderate bone structure
C) Large bone structure

Weight:
A) Slim to thin
B) Moderate to plump
C) Heavy, tendency to obesity

Skin:
A) Dry or mixed complexion
B) Tendency toward oily
C) Slightly oily

Joints:
A) Thin, small
B) Medium
C) Large

Perspiration:
A) Slight, little to no odor
B) Abundant, strong odor
C) Moderate, medium odor

Appetite:
A) Irregular
B) Strong, notices a missed meal
C) Constant, can comfortably miss a meal

Taste Preference:
A) Sweet, salty, oily
D) Bitter, spicy
E) Oily, hearty foods

Personality Tendency:
A) Intuitive and abstract
B) Judgmental and rational
C) Overly loving and giving

Memory:
A) Short, forgets easily
D) Average
E) Long term

Reaction to Stress:
A) Anxiety, fear, worry
D) Irritability, anger
E) Depression, complacency

Relationships tend to be:
A) Ever changing, be they with one or many people
B) Intensely passionate and explosive
C) Long term, stable relationships

Most Common Dreams:
A) Flying, nightmares, running
D) Anger, fiery, passionate
E) Sentimental, bodies of water

Spending Habits:
A) Spends quickly and impulsively
D) Spends moderately, with contemplation
E) Saves

Weather dislikes:
A) Cold, windy
B) Heat, sun
C) Cold, damp

Disease Dislikes:
A) Nervous system issues, general pains, arthritis, mental instability
B) Fertility issues, infections, inflammations, various skin disorders
C) Respiratory diseases, asthma, edema, obesity

Pulse type:
A) Rapid, snake-like
B) Strong, frog-like
C) Slow, swan-like

When you have completed the questionnaire, count the number of times you circled the letter A. List the number in the space provided. Do the same for letters B and C.

A)_____
B)_____
C)_____

Results of Quiz:
A = Air Constitution
B = Fire Constitution
C = Water Constitution

The letter with the highest number of answers determines your constitution. If two of the high numbers are identical, you may have two underlying or presenting constitutions. If all three of the numbers match, you may have all three constitutions equally distributed.

PULSE TESTING

WE CAN ACCESS A GOOD DEAL OF INFORMATION about a client by taking their pulse. The quality of the pulse tells us about a client's constitution. This technique offers the most direct and accurate result when done by an accomplished practitioner.

Connect synergistic points on the hand with a client's matching pulse points to feel the state of the client's constitution. Both the underlying and presenting constitution can be assessed through pulse testing.

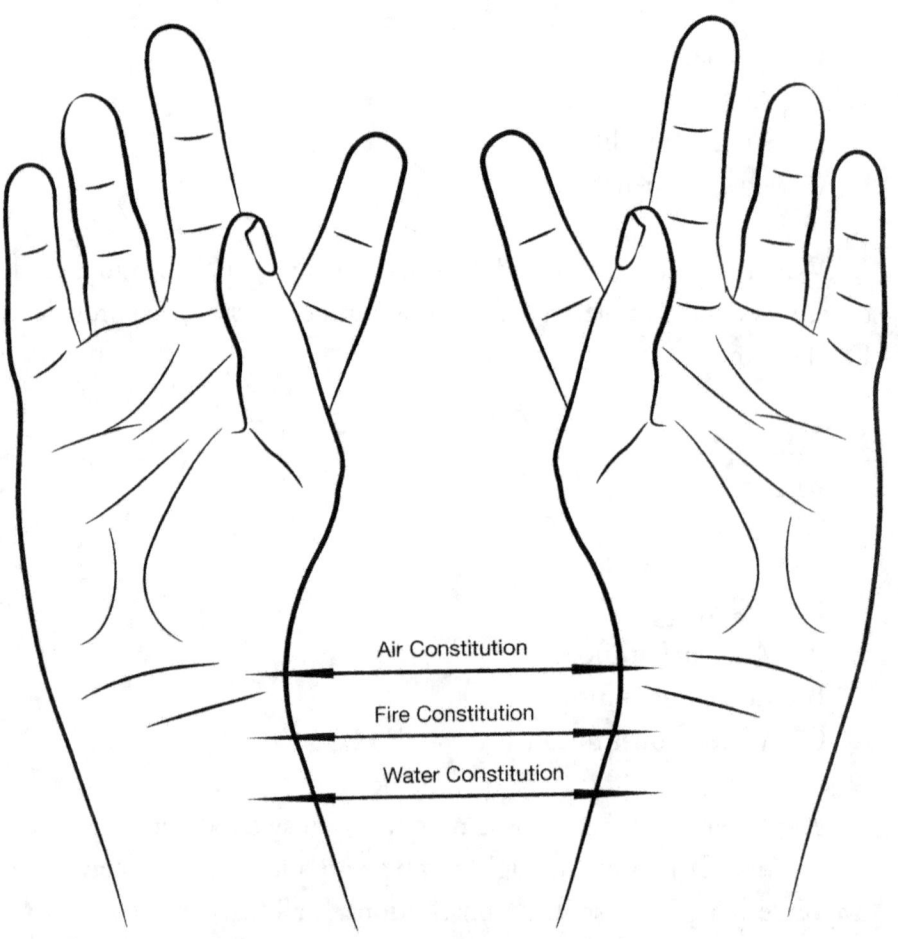

Pulse Testing

Place the index finger on the radial pulse below the flex in the wrist (i.e., two finger widths below the thumb root). The middle finger is placed just under the index finger, and the ring finger closest to the elbow. The practitioner's fingers lightly touch side by side.

The client's arm is relaxed, the elbow and wrist are slightly bent.

The tops of the practitioner's finger pads are softly placed and can easily read the pulse. Practitioner fingers are placed between the wide bone below the client's thumb and the thin bones in the middle of the wrist.

Finger pressure on the wrist is relatively firm at first, then gently lightens.

The first pulse the practitioner senses will be the presenting constitution type to be worked with.

- Fire Constitution is assessed by the middle finger. Quality of the pulse may be bouncy and intense.
- Air Constitution is assessed by the index finger. Quality of the pulse may be thread-like and erratic.
- Water Constitution is assessed by the ring finger. Quality of the pulse may be regular and deep.

Finding the Air Constitution may be difficult due to the weakness of a pulse. Assessing water and earth in a Water Constitution may also be difficult to find or read due to potential excess fat or thick skin.

Many other factors may cause inaccurate readings, so it is advised not to take pulses under certain conditions. For instance, it is not recommended that you take the pulse:

1. Following meals, exercise of strenuous work.
2. While nature is calling.
3. When suffering from fever.
4. During or after a bath or sauna.
5. After sunbathing, massage, while sitting near a fire.
6. Following a sexual encounter.

It is recommended to take the pulse between meals, while one is rested and after nature has called. With practice the pulse can be accounted for even during inopportune times.

Pulse of Individual Sephirah

He arranged in him all forms of higher mysteries of the world above and all forms of lower mysteries of lower world, all arranged in a person, who stands in the image of G-d, for he is called creation-hebrew-(kaf), the palm. [34]

—*Zohar,* Daniel C. Matt

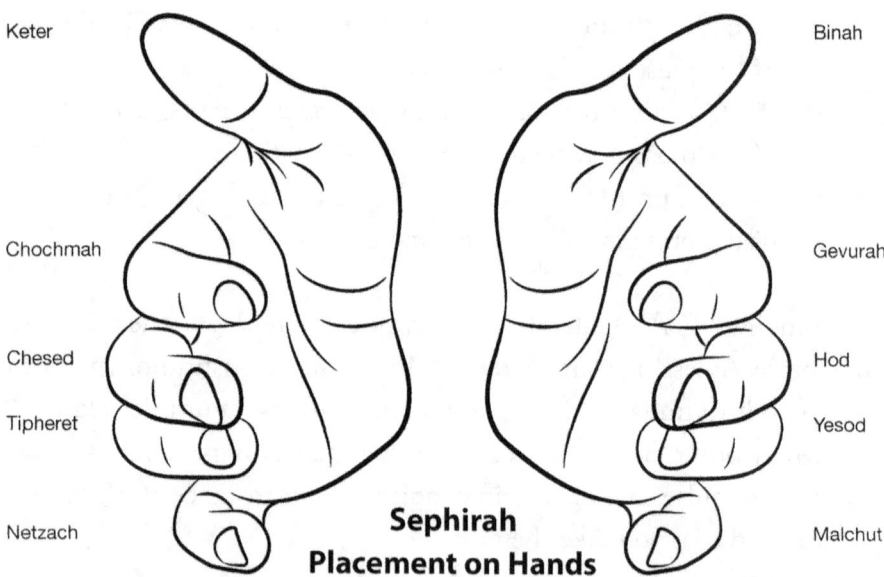

Sephirah Placement on Hands

We can determine the condition of each sephirah using pulse testing. This requires practice and an integral understanding of the esoteric anatomy of the hand and fingers. This practice gives us detailed information about treatment needs. The ToL reading that follows becomes a tool to fine tune the session rather than the driving force of it.

The entire body and the ToL within it is mapped out on our hand. Each finger represents a sephirah. Understanding which finger corresponds with which sephirah allows us to work with our fingers as healing tools.

Place the finger that matches the sephirah we want to assess on the client's matching sephirotic body point. Initially use moderate pressure and slowly lighten. Hold until the flow of energy is felt. Assess the quality of the pulse. This allows us to feel the state of the sephirah in their body.

This technique can also be done by placing the finger on the wrist. If working with the pulse on the wrist make sure the finger is on the pulse point that corresponds to the element of the sephirah. For instance, Tipheret corresponds to the element of air. When assessing Tipheret, we place out right index finger on the pulse point closest to the base of the client's thumb. This is the pulse that coordinates with the Air Constitution. Begin with firm pressure and slowly release. Allow the information about Tipheret to come to your right index finger.

We can also assess how a sephirah is influencing a constitution other than the one its element is associated with. For instance, to assess the state of the Sephirah of Tipheret in the Water Constitution of a person place the right index finger on the medial pulse. Apply firm pressure and slowly release. Allow the information about Tipheret to come to your right index finger.

Part III

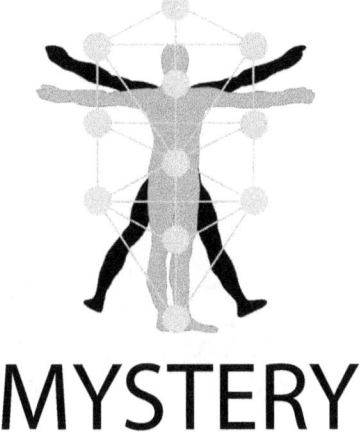

MYSTERY

Chapter 14

Angels

From here on, He makes His angels spirits... [35]

—*Psalms* (104:4)

ANGELS ARE FASCINATING. The very mention of an angel perks the ears. They seem to illicit a strong and diverse response in everyone. Humanity has maintained a belief or a knowledge of angels for thousands of years. To some they are thought of as companions, to others messengers or even souls of the stars. But why? What and who are the angels? Are they an anthropomorphic representation of natural forces, individual personas that interact with us in our daily lives or simply the illusion of fantasy? The answer is that they can be all or none of these.

Literature depicts angels in many different ways. KST focuses on older writings in order to gain better insight into the original intent behind the concept of angels. There were a limited number of angels described in this chapter to reflect the smaller number of angels discussed in ancient literature. However, there are an infinite number of possible angels.

During the course of human history more angels are continually referenced. Whether their presence is due to more angels being discovered, making themselves known or of our own making will be explored in the pages to come.

It is hoped that the information presented here will help enhance and expand the concept of angels within the KST community so that their influence can aid us personally and as healers.

Much of the ancient texts that contain the original descriptions of angels were written in Hebrew. The Hebrew word for angel is *malach* which translates as messenger or agent; it is as messengers that the malachim become angels.

In general, angels are messengers who are created to perform a specific task or combination of tasks. They exist for the duration of their task whether it be for a limited second or a limitless lifetime. Some are created with a thought or kavana (intention) and erased from existence along with the extinction of that thought or the completion of the kavana. Others are created to guide the life of a blade of grass or the life path of a person.

One angel cannot have two missions and angels have no way of knowing anything that does not pertain to their particular mission.

OLAMOT AND ANGELS

WITHIN THIS CREATION there are four primary olamot (worlds) that make up our universe. Each world represents a demarcation within the level of contraction of the infinite light.

As the infinite light descended from its source the frequency became slower and slower. The first and highest world to become manifest is called Atzilut (world of emanation). At this level, light is closer to the frequency of the original infinite light than the next World of Beriah (world of creation). Likewise, the third World of Yetzirah (world of formation) has a slower frequency than that of Beriah. The fourth Olamot World of Asiyah (world of action) has the slowest frequency. The World of Asiyah contains the physical world. Sometimes the four worlds together are simply called ABYAh.

This process of the sequential lowering of light or frequency that made the olamot worlds is referred to as the process of tzimtzum. The reason for the tzimtzum was so that creation could take place. Part of creation includes the angels. Each type of angel exists on the olamot world that best resonates with its particular frequency.

The archangels reside in the first Olamot World of Azilut. They have greater freedom of choice than other angels but not when compared to humanity. The sepharim, or fiery angels, reside on the second Olamot World of Beriah and can be likened to pure intellect. On the third World of Yetzirah the chayot hakodesh can be found along with the cherubim which are associated with pure emotion. On the fourth World of Asiyah, or the physical world, we find the ophanim who have a wheel like structure.

Knowing where each angel primarily resides is key to understanding what their purpose or mission is. Likewise, which angel you encounter will determine which olamot world they came from or which olamot world you are reading about, experiencing or assessing.

TEMPORARY ANGELS

TEMPORARY ANGELS EXIST FOR A SPECIFIC PURPOSE. Once that purpose is completed the angel will vanish from existence. Our own words, thoughts, expression or kavana create angels. Everything that moves with energy and intention can be an angel.

There are countless temporary angels at any given time. They are the messages and messengers that are meant for people, animals, plants and for all creation. Everything that contains a ToL contains life and anything that contains life will have at least one angel in attendance at any given moment. More than likely there is much more than one angel present for each ToL.

The temporary angels can appear very different depending on which of the four olamot worlds they were created on. This is because each category of angel was created or formed in association with a specific olamot world. Once we learn which angels go with which worlds, we are able to navigate our location in creation both in our studies and in the experience of dreams or spiritual occurrence.

By the middle ages the number of angels had become more plentiful and diverse. There were countless categories of angels depending on which clergy, theologian or philosopher was commenting. Today there are numerous encyclopedia-like texts that describe different details of angels. This chapter limits those types of details to the original four archangels and four categories of temporary angels. As will soon become clear, from this limited category, as many other angels as you wish to imagine can exist.

ARCHANGELS

The archangels of Azilut have individual names. Although they were created for a sole purpose just like the temporary angels, they have a limitless life span and can take on as many forms as needed for their particular mission. When they do take form, they are as souls to these forms. During such times it may appear that the archangel has multiple purposes and personas that are their own, however, it is the interaction of angel and form that creates this multifaceted appearance.

Archangels have freedom of choice but that choice is limited. This limitation is both because of the way they were created and also a product of being so close to Ein Sof or the Infinite. If we were as consciously aware of the light as the angels, there would be little to no desire for us to do anything other than the direct will of the infinite source of creation. This is because the closer we are to the light, the more we can see the bigger purpose of creation and understand the whys of it all. And if we understand the whys then we will choose the light every time. In order to have choice we stay in partial darkness.

More and more angels are mentioned as time goes on. There is room for all of them in our universe of infinite possibilities. Viewing each angel as a distinct persona can help us to identify with their message. But, we must remember that if we do identify with an anthropomorphic representation of an angelic force, we are doing it for our sake and not because it is necessarily the angels true nature. As KST practitioners we have to be extra careful not to see the angels as the form they present.

Archangel Seals

Archangel Michael

Archangel Gabriel

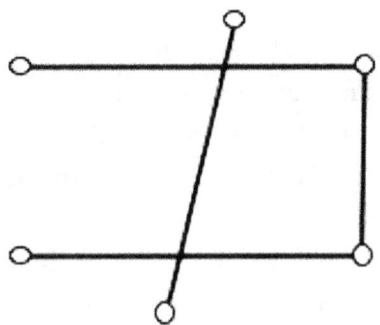
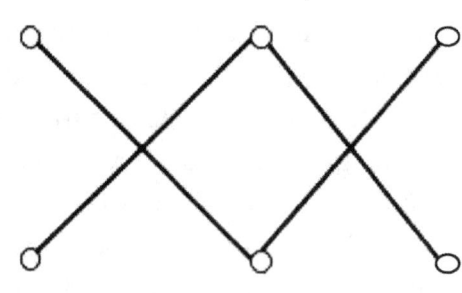

Archangel Uriel

Archangel Raphael

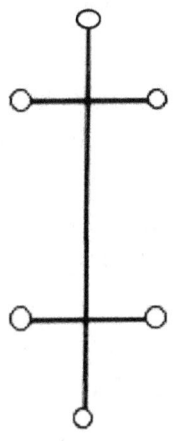
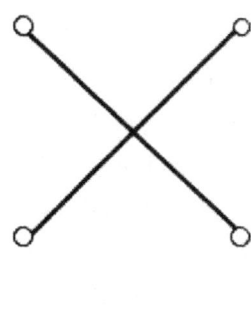

Archangel Michael

Making the clouds His chariot (Psalms 104:3) – Michael and Gabriel, who are clouds. [36]

—*Zohar,* Daniel C. Matt

Archangel Michael is associated with giving and mercy, the element of water, the right side of the ToL and the right arm of the body.

When in balance, this is a truly nurturing, loving, restful and peaceful energy. As such the Archangel Michael is closely linked with the Sephirah of Chesed, known for giving, hospitality and love.

Archangel Michael is one of the most beloved and popular archangels. He is a warrior angel that protects through patience and love. Over time many sightings, writings and events have taken place that were attributed to the Archangel Michael. Most religions and spiritual paths either claim the Archangel Michael as their own or recognize him as a legitimate presence. There is a strong scientific explanation for the archangels, including the Archangel Michael. This information is located in this chapter under the section titled, "The True Nature of Angels."

A good way to work with the energy of the Archangel Michael is to connect with the healing tools found after this section. They have a similar resonant frequency to the Archangel Michael. Since this archangel is associated with the Sephirah of Chesed, many of the same healing tools that apply to Chesed also apply to the Archangel Michael. Utilizing these tools with the correct kavana during a healing session can help amplify and direct the ohrim to help heal issues that involve Chesed, compassion or giving. They can aid in the release of hurts associated with being victimized, taken advantage of or feelings of depletion after giving too much. Conversely, the tools for healing listed below can help to release blocks that inhibit us from giving.

Attributes of Michael
- Anatomy - Right Arm
- Day - Sunday
- Color - Blue
- Direction - South
- Element - Water
- Essential Oil - Frankincense, Blue Tansy
- Gems - Amethyst, Aquamarine, Saphire, Lapis Lazuli, Turquoise, Clear
- Hebrew - ShMSh
- Metal - Silver
- Quartz, Fluorite, Geodes, Moonstone, Pearls
- Sephirah - Chesed
- Symbol or Seal - *(See illustration.)*

Archangel Gabriel

Archangel Gabriel is associated with strength, power and boundaries, the element of fire, the left side of the ToL and the left arm of the body.

When in balance, this is a focused, transformative, clear and just energy. As such the Archangel Gabriel is closely linked with the Sephirah of Gevurah, known for restraint, judgment and boundaries.

Archangel Gabriel is one of the most popular archangels. He is associated with magic, dreams and prophecy. Over time many sightings, writings and events have taken place that were attributed to the Archangel Gabriel. Most religions and spiritual paths either claim the Archangel Gabriel as their own or recognize him as a legitimate presence. There is a strong scientific explanation for the archangels, including the Archangel Gabriel. This information is located in this chapter under the section titled, "The True Nature of Angels."

A good way to work with the energy of the Archangel Gabriel is to connect with the healing tools found after this section. They have a similar resonant frequency to the Archangel Gabriel. Since this archangel is associated with the Sephirah of Gevurah, many of the same healing tools that apply to Gevurah also apply to the Archangel Gabriel. Utilizing these tools with the correct kavana during a healing session can help amplify and direct the ohrim to help heal issues that involve Gevurah, clarity or boundaries. They can aid in the release of hurts associated with injustice, crossing of boundaries or burn out. These healing tools can also help release blocks that inhibit us from standing firm in our own power or from expressing ourselves directly.

Archangel Gabriel is associated with the dreamtime. This is the perfect archangel to call upon for answers to the meaning of our dreams. Keeping a dream journal is an excellent tool for connecting with this energy.

Attributes of Gabriel
- Anatomy - Left Side
- Color - Red
- Day - Monday
- Direction - North
- Element - Fire
- Essential Oil - Myrrh, Orange, Cedar, Angelica, Marigold
- Gems - Ruby, Carnelian, Tiger's Eye, Amber, Citrine
- Hebrew - LBNH
- Metal - Gold, Copper
- Sephirah - Gevurah
- Symbol or Seal - (See illustration.)

Archangel Uriel

Archangel Uriel is associated with light, centeredness and revelation, the element of air, the central column of the ToL and the solar plexus or trunk of the body.

When in balance, this is an enlightening, mystical and core energy. As such the Archangel Uriel is closely linked with the Sephirah of Tipheret, known for beauty, inspiration, personal power and integrity.

Archangel Uriel is connected to the front of the body. Uriel has the most perfect light of all the archangels. This light mirrors the central sun of beauty that is Tipheret within us. Connecting with this light helps to bring enlightenment.

Uriel helps bring balance for the energy of the other archangels, especially Michael and Gabriel. There is a strong scientific explanation for the archangels, including the Archangel Uriel. This information is located in this chapter under the section titled, "The True Nature of Angels."

A good way to work with the energy of the Archangel Uriel is to connect with the healing tools found after this section. They have a similar resonant frequency to the Archangel Uriel. Since this archangel is associated with the Sephirah of Tipheret, many of the same healing tools that apply to Tipheret also apply to the Archangel Uriel. Utilizing these tools with the correct kavana during a healing session can help amplify and direct the ohrim to help heal issues that involve Tipheret, core identity, personal power and balance. This mesmerizing energy can help make sure our personal light and vitality is strong in order to ensure a sense of wellbeing.

Attributes of Uriel
- Anatomy - Trunk
- Color - Yellow, Rainbow
- Day - Friday
- Direction - East
- Element - Air
- Essential Oil - Sandalwood, White Lotus, Rose
- Gems - Clear Quartz, Diamond, Amethyst
- Metal - Platinum, Alloys
- Sephirah - Tipheret
- Symbol or Seal - *(See illustration.)*

Archangel Raphael

Walking on the wings of the wind (ibid.) - to provide healing to the world, and this is Raphael. [37]

— *Zohar,* Daniel C. Matt

Archangel Raphael is associated with healing and grounding, the element of earth, the lower part of the ToL and the spine within the body.

When in balance, this is a truly healing, supportive and sustaining energy. As such the Archangel Rafael is closely linked with the Sephirah of Malchut, known for protecting, grounding and abundance.

Raphael translates as, "G-d has healed." Archangel Raphael is charged with healing the earth. He is associated with physical healing and abundance. Archangel Raphael helps free us from our fears and issues around survival and gives us a sense of being supported and nurtured in the world. This energy corresponds to the back of our body, specifically the spine and nerves. There is a yogic saying, "healthy spine, healthy life." It is from the spine that nerves innervate the rest of the body. This creates an interconnection and inter-relationship throughout the entire body. There is a strong scientific explanation for the archangels, including the Archangel Michael. This information is located in this chapter under the section titled, "The True Nature of Angels."

A good way to work with the energy of the Archangel Raphael is to connect with the healing tools found after this paragraph. They have a similar resonant frequency to the Archangel Raphael. Since this archangel is associated with the Sephirah of Malchut, many of the same healing tools that apply to Malchut also apply to the Archangel Raphael. Utilizing these tools with the correct kavana during a healing session can help amplify and direct the ohrim to help heal issues that involve Malchut, healing and abundance. These healing tools can aid in establishing better health and both physical and financial stability.

Attributes of Raphael
- Anatomy - Spine, Nervous System
- Color - Rainbow
- Day - Wednesday
- Direction - West
- Element - Aether
- Essential Oil - Spikenard, Peppermint, Vetiver
- Gems - Hematite, Agate, Opal, Yellow Topaz or Serpentine
- Hebrew - KVKB
- Metal - Quicksilver, Aluminum
- Sephirah - Yesod

ANTHROPOMORPHISM

WE LOVE ANGELS. We want to connect with them. In order to do so, we generate anthropomorphic images for them that we can identify with, attributing characteristics, behaviors and motivation to the phenomena that are also relateable. Angels are sometimes depicted as having a human or animal form, as taking the shape of a wheel, or appearing in a combination of forms. These images can change over time. For instance, the original cherubim were characterized as fierce warriors that carried a mighty sword. Today a cherub is represented as a plumb baby with white fluffy wings. Did the cherubim themselves change over time or did we choose a different form with which to imagine them?

Whether the images or voices we associate with them are generated by the angels themselves or by our perception, anthropomorphic representations of angels are not accurate; they are for our benefit. Angels are messengers. We would likely miss the message if it came from an abstract force that did not communicate in a language we could comprehend. The forms angels take help us to hear their message.

By understanding that angels are messengers and associating their forms with their message delivery system, we can better conceive of and work with the energy of the angels.

Angels are forces more than anthropomorphic beings. Even when they do maintain creature-like or human-like form they have no physical functions and little to no individual will. The force that traverses the spiritual realms is what we call an angel. Even archangels may not act outside their express and singular function unless they were designed to do so for a specific purpose.

If angels only have one singular mission, then how is it that many seemingly do more than that? A comparison between the angel and a human soul may help bridge the answer. A human soul is also an energetic entity, and the same question could be asked about it. How can a single soul be involved in many tasks? But here the answer is obvious. The soul exists on different levels but is integrated by its association with a single body. It is not differentiated into many souls by its many tasks, because its association with the body allows it to remain an integrated whole.

Likewise, the archangels live forever while maintaining a singular function. Their association with a particular form provides for that singular task to complete itself in a myriad of ways.

TRUE NATURE OF ANGELS

Angels are forces of nature that relate to the elements. The four elements include air, fire, water and earth. In Kaplan's translation of the Sefer Yetzirah, he explains how these four elements describe what today's science calls the four forces of nature. The four forces are: the strong nuclear or pionic force (water), the electromagnetic force (fire), the weak nuclear force (air) and the gravitational force (earth).

The four archangels (Michael, Gabriel, Uriel and Raphael) correlate to the elements of water, fire, air and earth as a way to describe their basic character. Looking at this relationship from another perspective, these basic elements correspond to the scientific forces of nature and, therefore, those fundamental forces are also represented as the underlying, primal natures of the four archangels.

Water corresponds to the strong nuclear force that binds positively charged particles together. If only the strong nuclear force existed, all matter would be denser and heavier than a neutron star, where a teaspoon weighs about ten million tons. This would likely result in the universe becoming one big/small singularity or black hole. Water as the Archangel Michael is the strong nuclear force.

Fire acts as the electromagnetic force, through which all matter interacts. However, if this were the only force present, then all of the positively charged particles in matter would repel each other and nothing would interact. Fire as the Archangel Gabriel is the electromagnetic force.

Air correlates to the weak nuclear force which decides between water and fire. It is this force that allows light particles such as leptons and electrons to exist and create the balance needed with the electromagnetic and strong nuclear force. Air as the Archangel Uriel is the weak nuclear force.

Earth represents the gravitational force. This fourth force corresponds to the earth that provides a vessel for the other elements to interact. Earth is the reflection of their interaction. Earth as the Archangel Raphael is the gravitational force.

These four forces have been measured and described scientifically. However, information about their interactions, characteristics and overall natures, as well as understanding of their effects upon us and the universe around us, continues to unfold.

The connection between these forces and the archangels acts as a bridge between the scientific and the mystical. Viewing the angels from a scientific perspective offers us an alternative to the traditional anthropomorphic forms.

THE FIFTH ELEMENT AND THE ANGEL METATRON

Aether, also known as the quintessence or fifth element, was an ancient and medieval concept describing the material that permeates space. Aether is not discussed in Kaplan's writing, however, it is worth mentioning here.

The four forces described in the previous section represent atomic matter. That is the universe we know as the physical world of Asiyah. However, atomic matter only makes up three to five percent of matter in the known universe. The rest is attributed to dark matter and dark energy. Einstein theorized that the empty space between properties could be attributed to the concept of aether and recent scientific proposals have re-introduced aether as possibly representing dark energy and a fifth fundamental force.

Metatron is the name of an angel associated with a somewhat mysterious but also powerful and ubiquitous nature. He is often referred to as a greater presence than all of the other angels combined. One proposed etymology of the name would be made up of two Greek words, *meta* and *thronos* or "behind the throne," suggesting a hidden essence behind the created universe.

Aether would be the force behind dark matter and energy that represents 95-97% of the universe. We do not have a good understanding of what dark matter and dark energy is. For the purposes of the archangels, it is the vessel or womb of our universe. Therefore, dark matter and dark energy as Metatron are aether.

WORKING WITH ANGELS IN EVERYDAY LIFE

THERE ARE NUMEROUS WAYS to experience and work with angels in our everyday life. For instance, we might think of an angel when reciting an kavana, while contemplating meaning and manifestation, or in acting as a vehicle for the ohrim for the purposes of healing.

When thinking of an angel, begin by connecting to its greater glory as a force of nature, but refrain from defining its form. Then, allow it to take whatever form that will best serve the angel's message without being attached to the image itself. Should there be no form, just an abstract message, so much the better.

CONCLUSION

ANGELS HAVE BEEN A PART OF OUR LIVES, our history and our traditions for centuries. Over time, angelic names and personas have become more numerous and culturally accepted. But it is not the forces themselves that are shifting or unveiling. Rather, it is humanity that is molding angels, so as to better relate to them.

When seeking to connect with the messages of the angels, let go of the idea of an angel having a fixed form. Be open to receiving expressions of their authentic natures. A less specific image may represent a more direct communication. Still, if we need to anthropomorphosize the forces we know as angels so as to better relate to them, we are not doing anything wrong. The very form or image we envision may be an important component of our higher self's pictorial translation of the angel's essential message. The delivery of those messages is their task. As KST practitioners, receiving that guidance accurately, in order to fulfill our intention as healers, is ours.

Chapter 15

Color

By all colors, are refracted – a vision to gaze upon. [38]
—*Zohar,* Daniel C. Matt

COLOR GUIDES US ALONG our path in life. To learn the meaning and symbolism of color within the context of KST is to harness a deeply mystical tool for healing. All colors exist within us as the ToL (Tree of Life).

Our immersion in the world of color is profound and all-encompassing. We are like a fish in water who is the last to contemplate the water that it lives in. Likewise, we may never consider the color that surrounds us—it is simply a part of our day to day life, like the air that we breathe.

Our breath keeps us alive just as color affects our thoughts, behaviors and our environment. As we will learn later in this chapter, color's affect upon our being is both subjective in our reaction to it and objective in the measurable effects upon us.

Before we venture into the depths of color's mysteries, we must first consider what color is. We can then explore the healing capacity and spiritual meaning of color in our lives.

DEFINITION OF COLOR

The quality of an object of substance with respect to light reflected by the object, usually determined visually by measurement of hue, saturation, and brightness of the reflected light, saturation of chroma, hue. [39]

— Color | Define Color at dictionary.com

COLOR IS A GENERAL TERM that encompasses many facets. Taking some time to explore the fundamentals of color can help build a base of understanding for how we interact with it. Color in this chapter includes all the colors of the rainbow and the variations therein.

The variations and gradations of the rainbow colors are defined as "value" and "hue." These qualities of color each contain frequency that impacts the physical world around us and the internal world of our body and mind. As we break down these qualities of color, we can see them as part of the luminous tapestry of life.

QUALITIES OF COLOR AS PIGMENT

HUE IS THE DEFINING TERM for the name of a color or its frequency. When painting, a pigment is often used to apply color to a surface. In this case the pigment is a physical carrier for a substance that has the sought hue of a thing. It is the result of light bouncing off of the material substance. That substance causes the light to shift its frequency. As that shifted frequency passes through our eyes it is interpreted as the particular hue of the object by our brain.

The three primary colors in painting are red, blue and yellow. This means that those colors cannot be broken down into another hue, and mixing them in set combinations will yield all hues or colors of the rainbow. For instance, red and yellow combine to make orange; red and blue produce purple; yellow and blue yield green. Blending all hues of pigment together will result in a black hue or pigment and the absence of them will result in a white pigment. Hue can also be defined as "chroma."

Saturation refers to the intensity of a hue or chroma. The greater the saturation the farther the color is from the center of a color wheel. It is the expression of the bandwidth of light as reflected from a source. The more frequency exists in a bandwidth the greater the saturation of the color. If hue refers to the color itself, saturation would be the intensity of that color.

Value is the relative lightness or darkness of a color. Adding black or white pigment to a hue pigment will give it gradations in value. It helps to create our perception of form and space. For instance, orienting to the value of color as we learn to drive a car helps us to navigate traffic on a freeway. Mastering value as an artist can help to create spacial illusions such as three-dimensional perspective on the two-dimensional canvas.

Contrast of value helps us to assess the external world in order to see the separation of objects in space. Gradation of value suggests the object's mass and contour. In the previous example, the artist can use gradation of value to suggest the bright red of the apple and can use contrasting subtle hue behind the apple to add to its sumptuous definition until the two-dimensional treat looks good enough to take a knowledgeable bite of.

The world of primary hues as pigment comes into play when looking at the ToL from our physical perspective of Asiyah or the physical world. The ToL, as used in the practice of KST, utilizes these pigment relationships in chromotherapy and to differentiate among the sephirot. This is useful since we are physical beings in a world that expresses itself to us in varied hues.

Primary Colors of Pigment and Light

Visible light is an electromagnetic wave. The frequency of the wave will determine its color. In a vacuum, blue and red light will travel at the same speed (the speed of light). The color of light that our eyes perceive depends on its wavelength, ranging from shortest (violet) to longest (red).

The primary colors of light differ slightly from those of pigments. They are red, green and blue. This has less to do with the physics of frequency and more to do with the anatomy of our eye.

The retina of the eye contains receptors, known as rods and cones. Rods permit us to see black, white and grey and the cones show us color. Cones work in bright light, but not when it's dim, which is why we don't see colors at night or in low light. Together cones detect the three primary colors of light, but each favors a different response, depending on the light's wavelength. There is one cone type which responds more strongly to short (blue) light waves, another which more easily detects medium (green), and a third which favors long (red) light waves.

We perceive various objects as being different colors because of how they each absorb and reflect wavelengths of visible light. For example, a red rose has molecules that absorb violet and blue wavelengths of light, so that only red light is reflected from the flower. White objects reflect all the wavelengths of color; black objects absorb them all, reflecting no light.

Pigments and light each have their own set of primary colors and ways that they blend to form other colors. The primary colors of light are combined using what's known as *additive mixing*. A red light and a green light combine to help our brain perceive the color yellow. Where a red light and a blue light overlap, we will see magenta; an overlapping of green and blue produces cyan. If those three colors sound familiar, it is because magenta, cyan and yellow are the color primaries for computer printing (more on that in the next section). In the context of light, if all three primary colors are shown at once, we will see white.

Pigments (used for mixing paints) are combined using *subtractive mixing*. Primary colors for pigments are red, blue and yellow. Colors of paint each combine to absorb some colors (subtracting them) and reflect what remains. If you mix all the primary pigments together, all the light is absorbed, reflecting no light back to your eyes and you will see black.

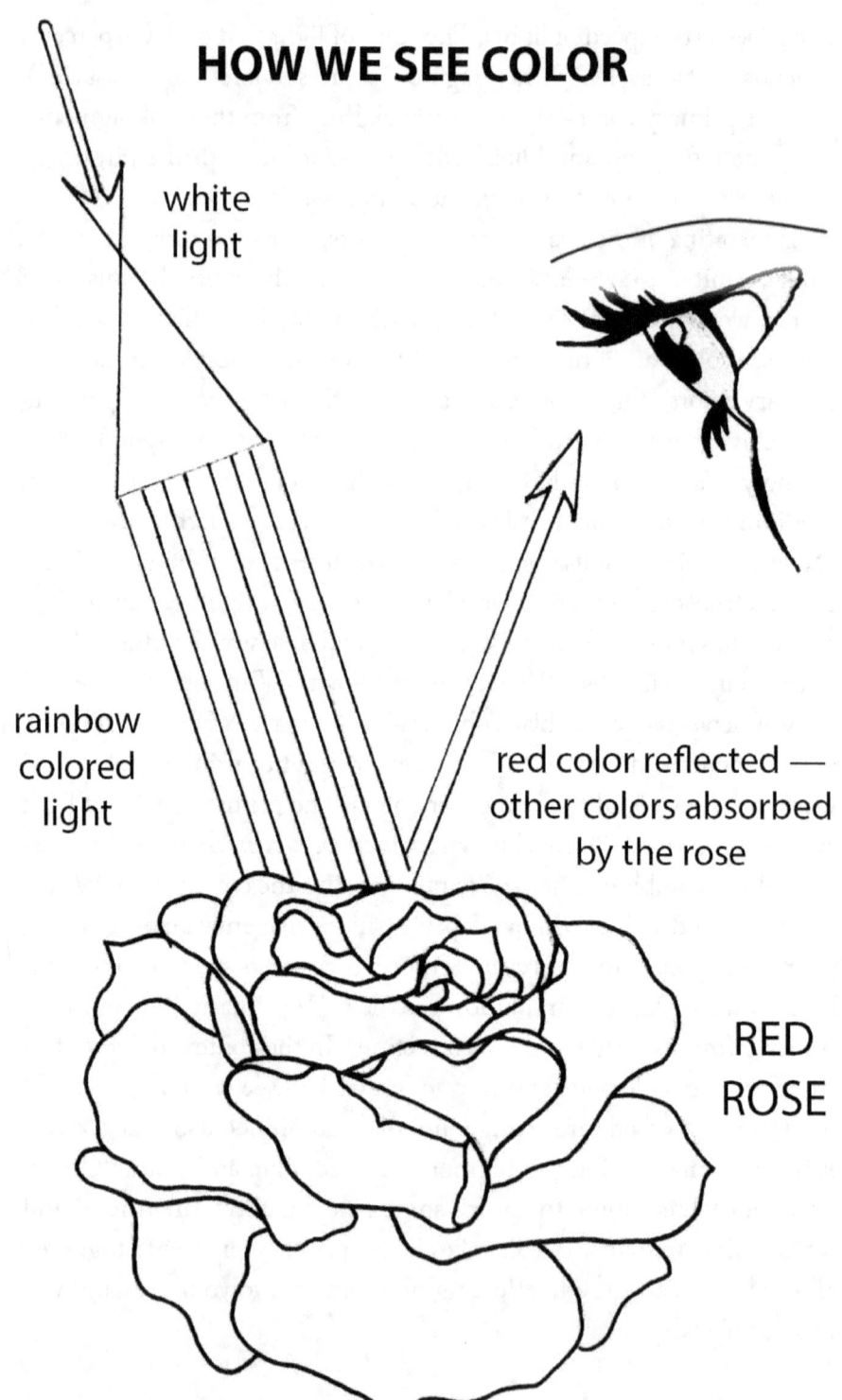

Language of Color

Color has a language. The alphabet of this language is made up of the primary colors, which combine to form the many words of this language as hues. We must get to know the primaries of both the physical pigment hues and the hues of light to be able to communicate congruently between the two worlds, where our experiences lie. Like memorizing the letters of a new language to create words, It just takes a bit of memorization of the primary colors of both pigment and light to visually articulate what is being said.

And God said, "Let there be light," and there was light. [40]
— Genesis (1:3)

The Big Bang, how scientists refer to the beginning of our universe, is believed to have been an explosion of energy and light. Both spiritual and scientific sources use the language of light to describe space and time, from both an earthly and a heavenly perspective.

Pigments are historically derived from earthly sources: minerals and gemstones, animal waste, insects, flowers and vegetables. Vermilion, the brilliant red of ancient Roman and Renaissance art, was originally made from the powdered mineral, cinnabar. The word derives from the Latin *vermis*, or "worm," a creature of earth. Artists throughout time have used the language of pigment to depict both earthly and heavenly subjects.

It is important to know the different primary colors for both light and for paints, as well as the ways they combine for our eyes to see color, not only for artists, but also for mystical and esoteric studies, such as Kabbalah.

The Zohar, one of the core texts in Kabbalah, describes the sephirot of Chesed, Gevurah and Tipheret as white, red and green or as blue, red and yellow, depending on the section being read and the intention. When the Zohar speaks of the different colors of the sephirot one must take into consideration the context.

The symbolism associated with a particular color could be interpreted to have an entirely different meaning than was intended if the differences between the primary pigment hues and light hues are not accounted for when translating ancient texts.

When accounting for the differences between light and pigment, the seeming inconsistencies in the Zohar's descriptions are revealed to be subtle differences in the language of color. The color palette for Chesed, Gevurah and Tipheret is actually the same; one is described using the alphabet from the higher frequency of light and the other from the lower frequency of earth. In both instances, the colors describing these sephirot can ultimately be broken down into yellow, red and blue. Green can be made by mixing blue and yellow. White can be made by either the absence of the colors for pigment or, when working with light, by combining all of them. In either instance all three colors are accounted for.

Why use different colors to describe the same thing? In the context of the Zohar the subtle variations relate to the message being offered, rather than a change in the color palette of the sephirot. Similarly, the Irish language uses two different words to describe the same hue of green, depending on the context: the word *glas* refers to the color of plants, *uaine* to the artificial green made by dyes and paints. *(Refer back to the illustration: ToL Ten Sephirot.)*

The ToL (Tree of Life) acts as a bridge between the world of physical pigment hues and those of light hues. In our work as KST practitioners, we have a similar function. By acting as interpreters, we help to create a flow of communication between the physical world of pigment and the worlds of light. Yet another link between light and matter was revealed with the introduction of computers.

Hue of Computer Printing:
Interpreting between light and pigment

Computer printing also acts as a bridge from light to physical matter. It is a perfect example of the sublime hidden within the mundane. In the context of KST, computer printing can be analogous to describing the sephirot, olamot worlds or angels as bridges from the ohrim to the physical world. These bridges have to interpret the information of one world so that the other can understand it and vice versa. The resulting translation becomes a language of its own, which acts as a gate between worlds. Each gate has a language engraved into its fibers. By learning the language spoken on a particular bridge in creation, we are accessing the keys to the gate between worlds. Think of it as having a Google Map of our universe that we could click to widen the view of, revealing the connecting roads, bridges, on-ramps and exits between two destinations. Our path toward whatever we seek is made that much easier to navigate.

The process of printing interprets light as pigment. It acts as a bridge between the additive world of light (such as a computer screen) and the subtractive world of the physical (ink on paper) as pigment. In order to interpret one to the other the bridge of computer printing needs to be able to translate one to the other. In doing so it has to use yet another set of primary colors. Just as each ascent or descent within the layers of the ToL requires knowing a whole new language, so too does the ascent or decent of frequency of color require a new way of interpreting it at each level.

Printing from a light source, such as a computer, is not just the mixing of physical pigments nor is it solely interpreting light hue. Rather, it has its own set of primary colors that are the language engraved on the gate at the bridge between physical pigment and light hue. If we were looking at color as the ToL, this gate could be likened to the veils that create either an illusory barrier or bridge between the olamot worlds.

In a way, both the printer and the KSTechnique® practitioner are a bridge for the universal healing light of the ohrim to be interpreted and channeled into the physical world. The ToL within us is the language engraved on the gate at the bridge that is our body. The difference being that the printer channels visible wavelengths of light from a monitor or screen whereas the KSTechnique® practitioner channels the universal healing light of the ohrim.

The computer printer interprets additive mixing of light and translates it into subtractive color mixing for the physical page. White light contains all of the possible colors of the rainbow. Light hue, interpreted as physical pigment, requires a reduction of those infinite possibilities. If a physical object reflects all of the possibilities of white light back to the eye the object appears white. If an object were to absorb all of this light, nothing would be reflected back to the eye and the object would appear black.

Printers use combinations of inks which act as physical filters, subtracting portions of the white light to produce various colors. The primary ink colors in printing are magenta, cyan and yellow. These printing primary colors are a bridge between the language of light (whose primaries are red, green and blue) and pigment (whose primaries are red, blue and yellow).

In the case of white light shining on a piece of printed paper, cyan ink will absorb/subtract red light from the white light and reflect both green and blue light, producing a turquoise color (which is cyan). Magenta ink absorbs green, reflecting red and blue light, which results in a purple hue (magenta). Yellow ink absorbs blue, reflects red and green, and appears yellow. To produce red, magenta and yellow combine to absorb the green and blue, reflecting and appearing red. By the same process, cyan and yellow appear green and cyan combined with magenta produces blue.

The differences between the primary colors of light, pigment and computer printing mirror the mystery of the worlds of light and world of matter being separated by a simple gate that, if opened, reveals that matter and light are one but just vibrating with different wavelengths. Without the printer and its interpretive primaries acting as a bridge of communication between the world of light and the physical world of ink, the resulting image on the printed paper would not be a congruent translation.

The primary hues in printing are the language spoken at the bridge between the worlds of light and the world of the physical. This bridge from light to pigment allows our eyes and mind to interpret and integrate light's messages in a physical form. More esoteric messages from the worlds of light can take years of study and meditation to translate. Luckily, printing an image of light from a monitor or screen is a simple process that requires little understanding of the science or design of printers. It only requires we see what we want to print and push a key; the printer does the rest. As KSTechnique® practitioners, it is our goal to be such a bridge for those who seek our help in translating the light of the ohrim into the physical realm of everyday life.

PSYCHOLOGY OF COLOR

COLOR IMPACTS US ON EVERY LEVEL of our being and its effects are often definable and measurable. Many of these effects are universal, however, these constants can also be influenced by things such as culture and personal experience. In addition to illuminating the human experience as a whole, this area of study provides insight into an individual's personality and behavior.

The study of the psychology of color involves understanding how color affects the mind. Colors affect us in such a way that we can sometimes not only see with our eyes, but also taste and feel.

Synesthesia is a rare neurological condition in which at least two of the senses are united. For example, some synesthetes feel, taste and/or hear color. These individuals experience certain sounds as having a color or particular letters or numbers as having an inherent hue. This ability, however, may be more universal than previously thought.

A number of neuroscientists hypothesize that all of us may be born experiencing the world as a unified whole, with the different sensory parts of the brain connected. These connections become blocked or trimmed as we mature. According to this theory, instead of five senses, we begin with one all-encompassing sense; at birth, our mother's voice might seem pink and have a scent.

Even after we mature, numerous studies have shown that color can affect how we taste, see and feel. The color of our mug can influence our perception of a coffee's flavor and intensity. Lighting in an office can affect productivity and mood. Color can influence both emotional and physical responses, from blood pressure and pulse to the perception of the weight of an object.

To define a color is to see it. To see a color is to be influenced by it.

One of the most interesting areas of research when it comes to culture and color has been assessing the process by which people define a color. According to some theories, prior to having a word to describe a color a person may not be able to consciously see it or be impacted by it. The eyes will see the hue but the brain will not process the information of the frequency associated with that color until it is defined in language. This may have occurred with most of the colors beginning with black and white and then going to all of the colors of the rainbow. In most cultures it is black and white that are defined first, then the lowest to highest frequencies whose order are: red, orange, yellow, green, blue and purple.

Like the universe unfolding in color segments as it cooled, the rainbow colors throughout human history would have unfolded as the verbal definition for these colors evolved. To not know the name of 'blue' might result in a method of describing using no color terminology at all. Once the rainbow hues have been seen and defined, or (according the aforementioned theories) defined and seen, there are numerous studies on the psychology of color to be explored.

For example, various studies with participants sampling from bowls of gelatin or water, which were tasteless but tinted with a variety of colors, have demonstrated the effects of our color associations on perception. Participants in this research described red as sweet like strawberry, yellow as sour like lemon and green as tart like green apples. Subjects in these tests were certain of the taste even after being told that the gelatin or liquid had no flavor added. In one experiment, a steak streaked with blue was perceived as having a rotten or unsavory taste, but only after the lights had been turned up and the color was fully visible.

According to multiple studies that focused on the connection between color and the perceived action of various drugs, including placebos, the color of drugs will tint our perception of their effects as well as their efficacy. For example, red pills would result in speeding the person up, blue was calming and good for sleep, yellow eased depression, green helped to subdue anxiety and white soothed pain.

There are cultural exceptions to some of these results. Italian men, for instance, associate the color blue with their national soccer team and the excitement of a game. As a result, blue has a stimulative, rather than a calming effect for them. Although the effects of color on the psyche may shift according to the cultural traditions, there do seem to be underlying consistencies across cultures. For instance, in Europe, in the US, and in Africa, black is the color of mourning. In contrast, throughout much of Asia white is the color of death.

For the purposes of KSTechnique, our cultural associations may tend toward the European since Europe's origins are more easily traced to Mesopotamia, the birthplace of western culture and KSTechnique, as found in traditional Kabbalah.

Color Keys

Black:
In balance: strong, defined, valuable
Out of balance: aggressive, hostile

White:
In balance: subdued, peaceful, innocent, angelic
Out of balance: lost

Red:
In balance: powerful, fertile, passionate, good boundaries, life enhancing, good judgment
Out of balance: aggressive, destructive, scary, violent, hatred, severe judgment

Orange:
In balance: sensual, warm, approachable, empathetic
Out of balance: lack of discernment, door mat

Yellow:
In balance: optimistic, joyful, centered
Out of balance: intrusive, ego based

Green:
In balance: peaceful nature, instincts, restful, embracing
Out of balance: decay, toxicity, overwhelmed

Blue:
In balance: spirituality, coolness, giving
Out of balance: cold, sadness, alienation

Purple:
In balance: fanciful, foundation, connection, intuition
Out of balance: fantasy, nightmare, sanguine, madness, disconnect

FREQUENCY

As stated previously in this chapter, visible light is an electromagnetic wave and the frequency of the wave will determine its color. Frequency is defined as the number of waves that pass a point during an interval of time (usually measured as one-second). A wavelength is the length of one complete cycle from crest to crest (highpoint) or from trough to trough (low point). Frequency is measured in units of these cycles per second. These units are known as *hertz*. *(Refer back to Electromagnetic Spectrum illustration.)*

We refer to the frequency of visible light as color. This rainbow ranges from red (at 430 trillion hertz) to violet (750 trillion hertz). Beyond the visible spectrum are lower frequencies, like radio waves (three billion hertz) as well as much higher ones, such as gamma rays (three billion billion hertz). The electromagnetic spectrum contains light waves of various frequencies, sizes and energies. A light wave's energy is related proportionally to its frequency. Radio waves have a small amount of energy. Gamma rays are dangerous to humans because of their great amount of energy.

The visible portion is only one-thousandth of one percent of the entire electromagnetic spectrum. Within the visual spectrum the color of red has the lowest frequency, lowest energy and longest wavelength. Orange has a slightly smaller wavelength and higher frequency and energy, continuing through yellow, green, blue, with violet appearing as the shortest wavelength, highest frequency and highest energy.

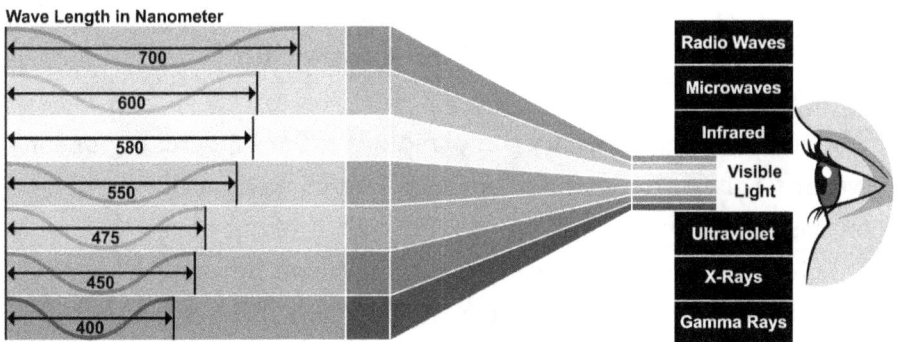

There is no judgment or faith around this concept. It is simply a wave measurement which defines frequency. Saying that red has a lower frequency only implies that it has a larger wave pattern. Saying that violet has a high frequency only means it has a smaller wave pattern. There is a vast range of wave sizes that make up the electromagnetic field.

Everything in the created worlds can be defined as different levels of frequency. Just as above mirrors below, so does the slower and larger frequency of our physical World of Asiyah connect to the smaller and quicker frequency of the higher World of Yetzirah. As with the colors of the rainbow, the function of one world is not better than another. Whether we are speaking of red as it relates to violet in the rainbow, or the World of Asiyah as it relates to Yetzirah, it is simply a matter of measurement of frequency that distinguishes them.

Measurements do not dispel the notion of mystery. Knowing the measurements and quality of the colors that make up a rainbow does not take away our awe of its beauty, nor does it hamper the psychological effects of its frequency on our mind and body. Rather, these measurements offer an understanding which can aid us in climbing or descending the ladder of self-realization on a conscious level. Many hidden mysteries lie beyond these measurements. And as the means to measure those mysteries are discovered and become mundane, there will be still deeper mysteries to reveal. The KSTechnique® practitioner uses both scientific and mystical tools to aid in the self-realization and healing process.

Frequency of Our Central Sun

The sun is our evolutionary companion. It is the Tipheret of our solar system's ToL. As the center of our solar system, it physically illuminates our vision and symbolically represents the joy of our being.

Our eyes allow us to see the world as color. But why do our eyes only see the one percent of the electromagnetic field called the visual spectrum? Is that sliver of the spectrum of color all that impacts us? Or is there a connection between the sun and our ability to only see the one percent that are the rainbow colors?

To operate and survive in our world, we need to know about objects: what they are and where they are. We've evolved to use that part of the electromagnetic spectrum that best accomplishes this goal. With some forms of electromagnetic radiation, short-wave radiation like X-rays or gamma rays for example, most objects are invisible. That is, the radiation passes right through them rather than reflecting off them to our eyes. Other forms of radiation, long-wave radiation like radio waves for example, would reflect off the objects to our eyes. But they would be so blurred as to be useless in any practical sense.

Our perception of the visible portion of the electromagnetic spectrum as color or hue is our physiological interpretation of the electromagnetic field. Our eyes cannot see beyond the rainbow colors and their combinations; however, we have built tools whereby we can measure these levels indirectly. Our body shows the effects of other parts of the electromagnetic spectrum. For instance, the invisible rays of ultraviolet affect the look and feel of our skin after we spend time in the sun, just as the heat of infrared can warm our food, light our rooms and keep us cozy on a cold night.

Our conscious perception of the world is limited to only a small fraction of reality. In the same way, our ability to see color is limited to one percent of the electromagnetic spectrum that is visible to the human eye. In Kabbalah it is said that we are only aware of one to ten percent of physical reality. This concept is mirrored in many other disciplines. Psychology has found that only a small percent of our behavior is conscious while the greater motivation behind our actions lies in the vast unconscious nature of our being. Physiologically we only utilize a small percentage of our DNA, leaving its greater potential in wait. Even in cosmology the atomic matter that makes up our visible universe only accounts for three to five percent of the matter and energy that is thought to exist. Our perception of ourselves, our world and the universe around us is veiled mostly in mystery.

Living in partial awareness helps us feel separate from the whole that is truth. This illusion of separation gifts us free will and that freedom offers us opportunities for unparalleled experience and growth. As we seek entry into the mysteries around us, we begin to become conscious within those hidden realms. Like the petals of a flower bud opening to the sun, we unfurl our realization into light, entering a path toward a greater conscious awareness and a growing understanding of the vast connections and oneness that is our true nature.

It is almost impossible to lose sight of our purpose, our center and our being as we traverse the universe. This center is mirrored by our Sun, not because the Sun is the center of the universe but because it is the center of our solar system. As residents of that system, that is where our eyes and our cycles have been focused. And what better way to aid in helping us survive than for our eyes to be most accustomed to interpreting the frequency of light that is most predominant on Earth. Our Sun's yellow is Tipheret as the center of the ToL (Tree of Life). It is the beauty at the core of our being. Yellow is located at the very center of the visual spectrum. The rest of the colors of the rainbow and their combinations are arrayed around it, just as the planets of our solar system and their respective moons are configured around our Sun.

If we look at yellow on the electromagnetic spectrum and then move our gaze to the left, we see yellow light become orange and then move into red as wavelengths get longer and frequencies get lower until they become invisible to our eyes at infrared. To the right of yellow the wavelengths get shorter and the frequencies higher until yellow becomes green, then blue, then violet. If we continue to measure in this direction, the shorter wavelengths and higher frequencies become ultra violet and gamma rays, which our eyes also cannot see. *(Refer back to the Electromagnetic Spectrum illustration.)*

The visual spectrum of the electromagnetic field is the portion that our sun predominately emits. The yellow light of the Sun is the very center of this rainbow. As such, it vibrates in the middle range of the spectrum that is visible to our eyes. Our ability to see yellow and the frequencies that are a bit lower and higher than yellow are a highly adaptive manifestation. This allows us to see the frequencies that most impact our physical environment. It is the center of our visual universe that we have oriented to since the dawn of our human creation.

Tipheret as the Central Sun of ZA

The Sun is to our solar system as Tipheret is to the ToL.

ZA (Zeir Anpin) is the central part of the ToL (Tree of Life). It is comprised of the Sephirot of Chesed, Gevurah, Tipheret, Netzach, Hod and Yesod. ZA translates to "small face" and is representative of our emotional world. Each of these six sephirah is associated with a particular color. Together, the sephirot contain all the colors of the rainbow.

Each of the sephirah that make up ZA is a holographic world unto itself. Through time, direction and experience, these sephirot have connected in order to better facilitate purpose in our physical world. From our perspective, each is associated with its own direction in space, frequency as color, and a myriad of other distinctions. Yet all are connected and are ultimately one, just as the universe and beyond are one. Apart they are tangential facets of a whole. Together they help create the very structure of our spiritual, emotional and physical worlds that offer us the experience we call life.

Tipheret, the sephirah of beauty, is represented by the color yellow in KST. Like our own physical Sun is the center of our galaxy, and just as the color yellow is surrounded by all the colors of the rainbow on the visual spectrum, Tipheret maintains its place at the center of the sephirot of ZA (Zeir Anpin). The Sun's bright yellow glow sits symmetrically between the lower frequency red side of the rainbow and the higher frequency blue side, just as the red of Gevurah and the blue of Chesed balance above and below, equidistant from Tipheret.

CHAKRA

THIS CHAPTER HAS DISCUSSED RAINBOWS and ZA, but what is a chakra? A chakra is a similar energy center of the body as that of a sephirah in the ToL within the body. The first written mention of chakras is found in the Vedas or holy books of India. They are mentioned along with Ayurveda (East Indian medicine), Yoga and Vastu (East Indian Feng Shui). The seven primary chakras are Muladhara (root chakra), Svadhisthana (sacral chakra), Manipura (solar plexus), Anahata (heart chakra), Vishuddha (throat chakra), Ajna (third eye), and Sahaswara (crown chakra). They are each connected to a different gland in the body, associated with a different color and have a different purpose. There are 42,000 chakras. However, it is these seven that are the most well known.

If you web-search the connection between chakras and the ToL, most results will show a horizontal breakdown of the connections. Although not inaccurate, this common way to view both the ToL and Chakras (Ayurveda) represent what can be described as the common or "revealed" understanding of both areas of study. There are two less conspicuous or "concealed" ways to see these connections.

The difference between these revealed and concealed observations can be compared to the common classroom demonstration of looking at the refracted image of a pencil sitting in a glass of water. At first glance, bending light rays can trick our eyes into seeing part of the pencil as wider and crooked, when it is actually slender and straight. But, once we learn about how light travels within different mediums (in this case, air vs. water), by simply moving the pencil to the center of the glass we can discover the true shape and form of the pencil behind the surface illusion. So, if understanding the concept of refraction can help us observe the concealed truth of a half-submerged pencil, what are the diagrams that connect the sephirot and chakras beneath the surface?

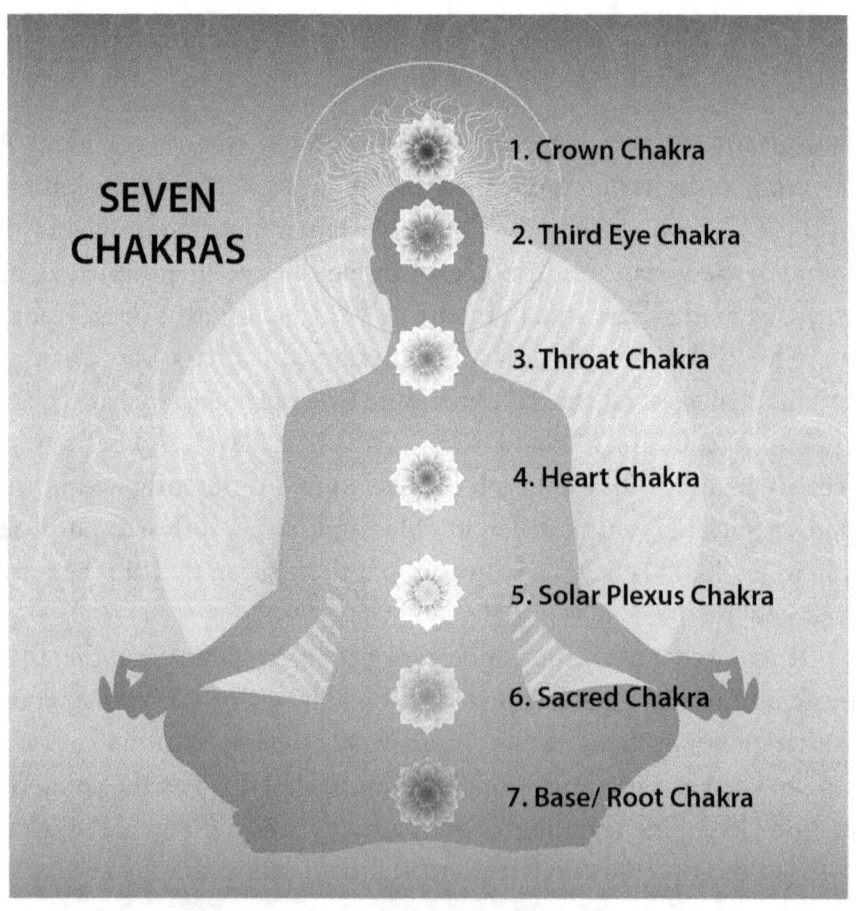

ZA, Chakras and the Rainbow

Two parts of a pencil can appear to diverge when observed within two different mediums. Similarly, ZA and the chakras can be seen as parts of the same mystery within different philosophies.

ZA is made up of the Sephirot of Yesod, Hod, Netzach, Tipheret, Gevurah and Chesed. They are the emotional attributes or *middot*, found in the ToL on the level of Yetzirah, the level just above our physical World of Asiyah, as found in Kabbalah. Like the chakras, ZA contains all of the colors of the rainbow.

The seven main chakras are energy centers found in the body. They represent the emotional attributes within the chakra system on the astral plane, or plane just above our physical plane, as found in the Vedas of India. The seven major chakras are represented by the colors of the rainbow.

Zeir Anpin and the seven chakras each comprise the emotional attributes of their respective systems, found on the same levels of existence but with different names. Both are connected to the frequencies of the rainbow and can be located within the body. The subtle differences, such as exact location in the body or attributes found outside of the body are minimal and easily explained with further study. First, let's explore the origins of what they share.

The story goes that thousands of years ago, during the time of Abraham, the trade routes between Mesopotamia and India were open. That is what is meant in Genesis when it says that Abraham sent some of his sons to the East with many gifts, including the spiritual gifts of Kabbalah. Whether this was Abraham as a person, patriarch or collective culture, it was then that certain secrets of Kabbalah found their way to India. This influence can be seen in the Vedas, which began to be written during that period. Those texts eloquently incorporated the tantric ideology of India at that time with Kabbalistic philosophies. Interestingly, ancient Mesopotamian illustrations exist from this time period that appear to depict yoga asanas, showing that the influence of culture went both ways.

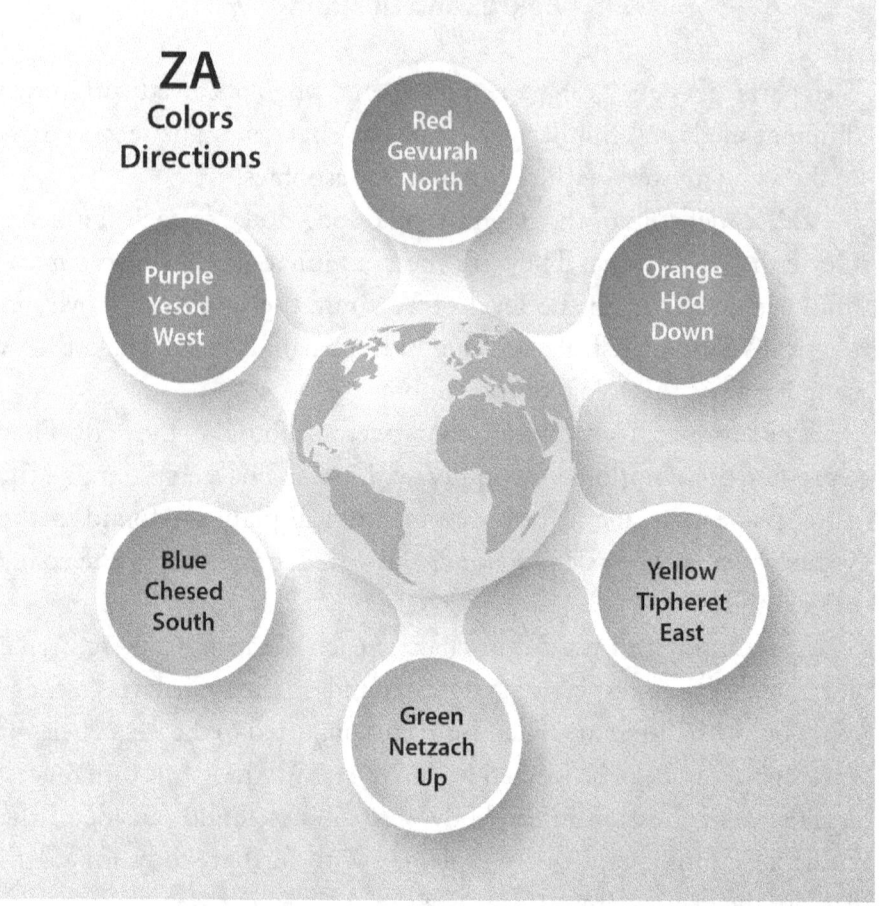

Like the half-submerged pencil, whether one contemplates the body by studying the chakras or ZA, each can be viewed as different aspects of a greater whole. We are all one. We exist on a unified plane as one. But the world of the rainbow appearing as both ZA and the chakras is one of duality, where we can experience individuality among a magnificent illusion of differences.

Are the Sephirot and Chakras the Same?

The sephirot are the building blocks of the ToL. In KSTechnique® the sephirot are read as energy centers in the body similar to how the chakras are read in the body. However, the sephirot also form the building blocks for the macrocosmic universe as a whole as well as any microcosmic universes unto themselves. They are a portal of contained and transmitted energy.

When looking at each sephirah and chakra from the perspective of the rainbow, we see the beautiful presence of the visual spectrum from red to violet with our Sun's yellow in between. Each of the sephirah of ZA and each primary chakra is associated with a frequency of color in the rainbow. Additionally, the sephirot of ZA are also connected to directions in space and time.

In order to gain a better understanding of how ZA directly correlates to our life experience, we can first take a look at its connections to the directions, and their associated colors, as frequency. They are:

Chesed - blue - south
Gevurah - red - north
Tipheret - yellow - East
Netzach - green - up
Hod - orange - down
Yesod - purple - west

(Refer back to the illustration: ToL Ten Sephirot.)

Upon further reflection on our orientation to time, space and frequency, a pattern can be seen to form. Just as we are oriented to the Sun's electromagnetic frequency as the center of our visual world, let us consider how we are oriented in space, beginning with the form of the familiar two-dimensional maps where north is up, south is down, east is to the right and west is to left.

As the journey continues, we can now explore hidden connections; one of color as energy, and a map to our place in spacetime.

Seven eyes of YHVH are the eyes of the community, seventy members of the Sanhedrin.[41]

— *Zohar,* Daniel C. Matt

Begin by holding a shoe string, or by imagining yourself holding a shoe string. Pin the beginning of the she string at the north point of the two-dimensional map. Allow the shoe string to fall in a clockwise manner so that it curves around the entirety of the map's directions until the shoe string completes its journey around the circle such that the end of the shoe string meets the beginning.

The end is embedded in the beginning.[42]

— *Sefer Yetzirah,* Ayreh Kaplan

Take a red marker and color the beginning of the shoe string in the north red. Now go to your right and color the section of the shoe string's path that is between north and east an orange hue. Color the east section of the string yellow, the curvature between east and south green, the south blue and the west a vibrant purple. Next, write the names of the sephirot next to their associated colors. The diagram and shoe string should look something like the following illustration:

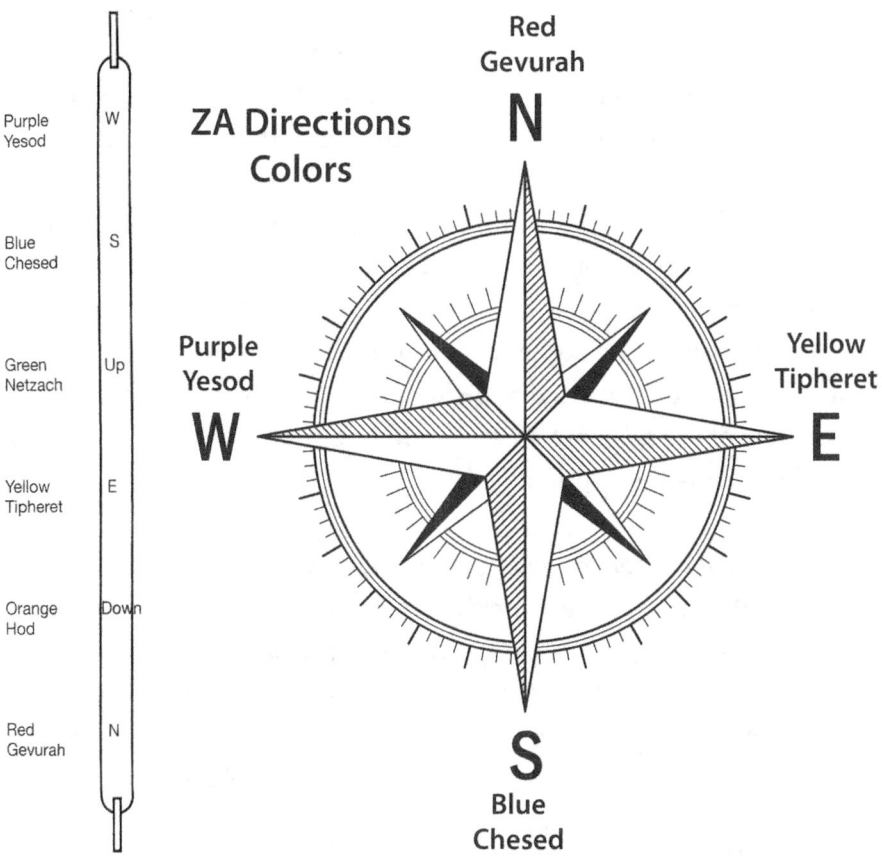

The sephirot will align with their rainbow colors. The placement of Hod is in between Gevurah and Tipheret, as it shows the healing energy descending toward Chesed from above to below. This shows Chesed being at the bottom when compared to the Supernal Triad and that descent is needed in order to ascend to its great height. The green of Netzach flows between Chesed and Tipheret ascending from below to above. Netzach and Hods placement depict their function as channels for our ascent and decent on the ToL.

Both Netzach and Hod have the power to connect with Malchut directly or channel their energy through Yesod the way the other sephirot do. Therefore, their placement surrounds Tipheret and not Yesod on the two-dimensional map. This represents their autonomy from the channel of Yesod. Netzach and Hod are the sephirot of prophecy.

One of their many gifts is to facilitate the flow of the other sephirot from above to below and below to above, should the channel for their energy merit it. When prophecy is cut off it is a reflection of our lack of connection with the higher realms. It is then that Netzach and Hod will surround Yesod on the two-dimensional map and cause discord in the flow of the rainbow. That is similar to our condition today. This map shows how they optimally function.

Seven supernal eyes, corresponding to the mystery that is written: Yours, O YHVH, (241b) are (Hebrew) (gedullah), greatness (Hebrew) Gevurah), power: (Hebrew) (tif'eret), beauty; (Hebrew) (netsah), victory; (Hebrew) (hod), splendor-yes, all that is in heaven and on earth (1 Chronicles 29:11). The one completes every side.[43]

—*Zohar,* Danial C. Matt

By shifting our perspective beyond the two-dimensional one, a hidden connection has begun to peek out from behind the seven horizontal rainbow slices found via a cursory internet search of the relationships between the chakras and ZA. The concealed begins to reveal itself further in the uncurling of the string (now wound around the directional map of ZA) into a straight line.

How?

Take hold of the end of the string at the point where it is colored purple. Unfurl it as you pull the string up vertically into a straight line. Place the string with the red side down and the purple side up to see the pattern of the chakras revealed to be that of the sephirot. Recall the refracted image of a half-submerged pencil: by reorienting the string we have effectively moved the pencil to the center of the glass. Two seemingly divergent systems can be seen as one when observed from a different perspective.

Placing the colored string onto a two-dimensional map demonstrates how the associated directions of ZA coordinate with our orientation to the world and how we navigate in the world. When we then uncurl the string into a straight line, with purple at the top and red at the bottom, this perspective reflects how we are created to be a bridge between heaven and earth.

The chakras follow this pattern of ZA stretched into a line. The purple/indigo of the Ajna Chakra is at the top and the red of Muladhara Chakra is at the bottom. The chakras are attached to the physical body. They begin at the spine and are associated with a gland. Each chakra then spirals outward and reflects a more vibrant color in the astral field, Body of Yetzirah or emotional body. These chakras describe the physical manifestations of ZA. They are rooted in the physical body of Asiyah and spiral outward to Yetzirah, connecting us to our aura, avir or worlds.

Both the sephirot and chakras look similar when viewed from the Body of Yetzirah or Astral Body. But their origins are different. The chakra is an emanation of the physical body whereas the sephirot are emanations from the original source of creation.

Think of the sephirot of ZA collectively as a door and the chakras as keys to that door. Where the chakras are rooted in the body, ZA is rooted in the source of creation above. The spiral energy centers of the chakras in the body are as angels or vessels that refract the original light source into the rainbow of human attributes.

The emotions are said to reside in the World of Yetzirah. The astral field is the emotional body just as the Body of Yetzirah in KST is the emotional body. Astral, Yetzirah, emotional body, chakra and the sephirot of ZA are different terms from diverse sources that all lead to the same place in time, space and emotion. The emotional body of the astral field and Yetzirah is where all the colors of the rainbow associated with the chakras and ZA reside as one.

It is popular to reference someone's aura as a certain rainbow color. However, like our ability to only see a small fraction of the electromagnetic spectrum, this aspect of the sephirot as ZA and the chakras is only a fraction of our avir as a whole. Greater detail of this can be found in chapter eleven of the first book.

Merkabah, ZA, Chakras and the Body

There is one more concealed connection to go.

The merkabah is a three-dimensional representation of ZA. In two dimensions it is the six-pointed star. It is a vehicle for soul traveling.

Go back to our two-dimensional map of the Earth. Draw a six-pointed star over the map. Make sure each point of the star connects with a direction. This is the two-dimensional representation of the merkabah. This is how ZA, chakras and our bodies connect in dimensional space time.

Details of the merkabah will be covered in the next book. For now, it is mentioned here, and in the chapter titled, "Soul Traveling," where it is a part of the KSMT meditation at the end of that chapter.

THE RAINBOW AND YOU

IF YOU HAVE MADE IT TO THIS PARAGRAPH, through the preceding labyrinth of color and connections, may you now take a breath, close your eyes and enjoy the rainbow and sacredness that is you.

Chapter 16

Soul Traveling

BRINGING CONSCIOUS AWARENESS TO THERAPY AND TO OUR LIVES THROUGH THE ART OF SOUL TRAVELING

A human being is a part of the whole, called by us 'Universe,' a part limited in time and space. He experiences himself, his thoughts and feelings, as something separate from the rest—a kind of optical delusion of consciousness. This delusion is a kind of prison for us, restricting us to our personal desires and affection of a few persons nearest to us. Our task must be to free ourselves from this prison by widening our circle of understanding and compassion to embrace all living creatures and the whole of nature in its beauty.[44]

—Albert Einstein

WHAT IS SOUL TRAVELING?

SOUL TRAVELING IS THE MOVEMENT of our soul into a more universal experience. This may take on a variety of forms. When we are learning to soul travel, we are taught to quiet our mind. When this is accomplished, we may see a flicker of light between our brows, then hear a distant sound at the back of our head. That sound comes from the inner ear. In Kabbalah this relates to the invisible Sefirah of Da'at as an externalized aspect of the Sephirah of Keter.

The practitioner focuses on this distant sound, for it is the frequency in which we will travel during meditation. In many cases we are catapulted into what appears to be space, with stars, galaxies or planets all around. This is usually followed by a sense of peace and union with all creation. As previously mentioned, this experience of a starry world relates to the bridge between the Olamot Worlds of Asiyah and Yetzirah, the Shechakim, or skies.

But have we actually traveled anywhere? The answer is yes and no. The soul exists on all olamot worlds at once, just like the holographic universe described in physics. What may feel like movement or travel is actually our soul's awareness coming into agreement with fixed states and conditions that already exist in time and space. For instance, the soul's aspect on Asiyah is called Neshamah, and its aspect on Yetzirah is called Ruach, but they are the same soul. What we perceive as movement is our consciousness shifting its focus onto different parts of the same soul—a soul that already exists on each of these levels.

The beauty of this is that the soul can never actually get lost, as it has not physically traveled anywhere beyond where it already is. Soul traveling is about a shift in consciousness rather than a shift in a specified time and space positioning.

KSMT

KSMT (KS MEDITATION TECHNIQUE) is a meditative technique practiced in KSTechnique® that aids the practitioner or client in achieving a more unified, peaceful or transcendent state of consciousness. Often called soul traveling, this experience can be entirely liberating, rejuvenating and transformative. An extreme experience of it is found in many NDR (near death) accounts. This technique helps achieve those sublime states without the need of extremes.

It is one thing to intellectually grasp that the universe is all connected and quite another to have a personal experience of that truth. Intellectual understanding provides a sense of faith. A direct experience of universal oneness as a state of consciousness brings a level of knowledge that becomes an inherent part of the practitioner or client.

The experience of soul traveling, unification, NDE (near death experience) or similar ecstatic experience is not an end in itself, but it does aid in an expansion of consciousness often necessary for personal development and awareness. The more we expand our consciousness, the more we can understand the experiences of others.

Remaining grounded during any of these explorations into creation and healing is imperative to give us a foundation to work from. Understanding the nature and purpose of the physical often aids in a sense of grounding while exploring higher realms and a higher purpose.

This experience of grounded universal connection enables us to be fully present in the moment, in our life and in our practice. This technique can be an effective and meaningful tool for the purposes of healing as well as self-discovery.

The physical world and our physical body are merely a slowed down frequency or reflecting vessel for the higher realms. Our body is a physical manifestation of these nonphysical realms, which vibrate at a higher frequency. In this sense the physical becomes a slower frequency of a quicker one.

THE INVISIBLE SEPHIRAH OF DA'AT

Although we initially study the ten sephirot, there is an eleventh called Da'at or the invisible sephirah. Its quality is that of knowledge. Its nature is connected to the entire universe. In biblical lore it is known as the Tree of Knowledge.

Da'at is the invisible sephirah of knowledge. There are no colors or elements associated with Da'at. There is only the deep knowing of everything that exists. To become aware of Da'at is to approach the

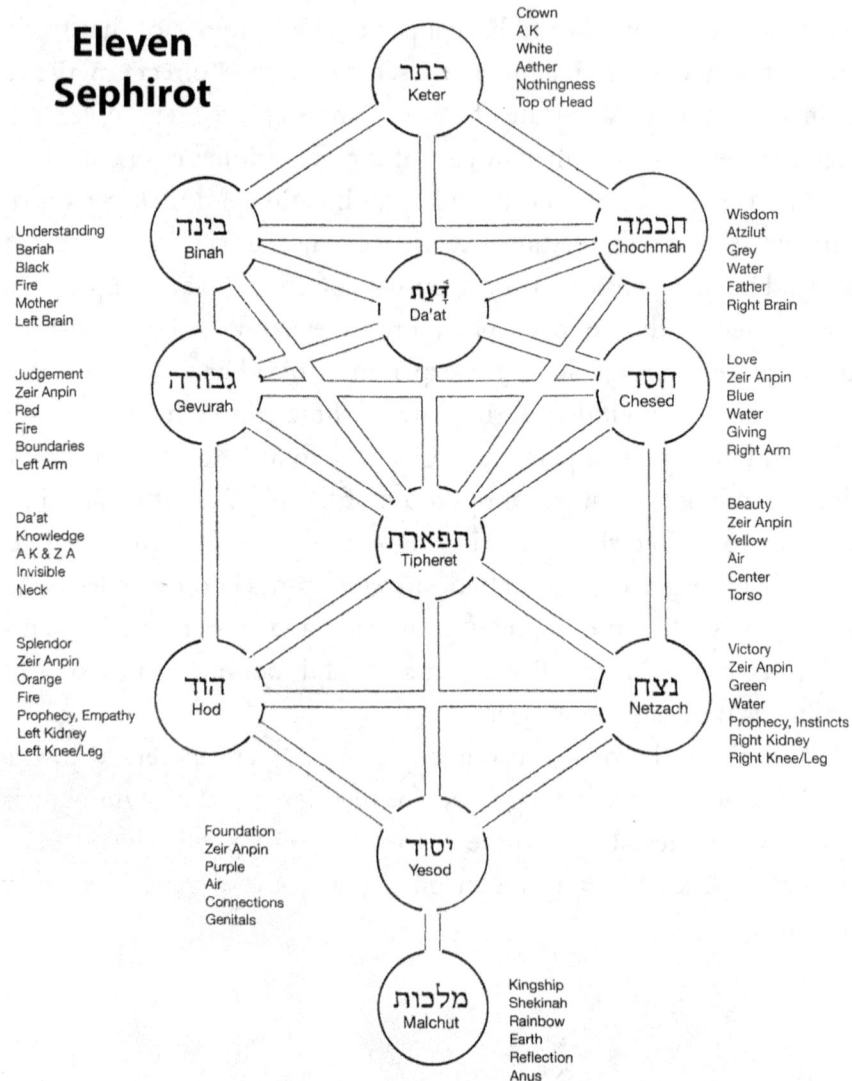

unification experience. To connect with Da'at is to connect with the universe as a whole. It's that aha moment when everything makes sense as a pattern in the cosmic play of things.

Da'at is located in the central column of the ToL (Tree of Life) below Keter and above Tipheret. It is just below the supernal triad of Keter, Chochmah and Binah. Keter becomes Da'at when it lowers its frequency within creation.

The corresponding location in our physical body is the neck area. Bodyworkers can access Da'at by massaging the area around the occiput at the back of the head and neck. KST practitioners can perform a KSH or KS hold protocol as shown below. Psychotherapists can work with a bodyworker to do these holds if appropriate and statutes permit, or they can do the distance healing technique found in chapter ten using the KSH protocol as a framework. The occiput is the area that helps us access the unification or soul traveling experience.

KSH Protocol for Soul Traveling

1. Stand beside supine client. With palms up, place one hand under the client's occiput and other under their sacrum. Hold kavana until you feel the energy flow. It will feel like a pulse between your hands. Gently release the hold.
2. Sit at the head of the client. Place both of your hands, palms up, under the client's shoulders until you feel a pulse. Then, bring both hands together under the client's occiput until their head rests comfortably in both palms. Hold until you feel a pulse. Release.
3. Cradle the back of the client's head with your thumbs at KT and four other fingers evenly spaced on the temporal region, with ears resting between them until you feel a pulse. Release.
4. Place one hand beneath the neck while the other rests on the forehead until you feel a pulse. Release.
5. Continue to place your hand on the client's forehead while you move the other hand unto the client's upper decollete. Hold until you feel a pulse. Release.

The KSH protocol is meant to help balance the supernal triad by bringing it into balance with the rest of the ToL (Tree of Life) within the body. In this way the body is strengthened so that it can hold a greater flow of the ohrim. This protocol is also found in chapter ten.

Lurianic Kabbalists say that the vessels of the original sephirot were shattered by the overwhelming light of creation. This process mirrors the Big Bang theory and supersymmetry of today's science. By coming closer and closer to that original state of oneness we enter into the world of tikkun or rectification, whereby these vessels are restored until they are strong enough to contain the light.

On a personal, microcosmic level, this process of rectification and healing assists us in fulfilling our potential in life. Healing ourselves in this way helps the world on a practical, macrocosmic level. When we strengthen our own vessels, the vessels of the universe are also strengthened, just as when the individual cells in our body are repaired and strengthened, so does our overall health improve.

Qualities associated with Da'at are found below. They can be added to the protocol script for the ToL reading found in chapter ten:
- Da'at
- Sephirah of Knowledge.
- There are no colors or elements associated with Da'at.
- It's about the unification experience. To connect with Da'at is to connect with the universe as a whole. It's that aha moment when everything makes sense as a pattern in the cosmic play of things.

CMBr

THE COSMIC SOUND HAS BEEN HEARD by countless individuals, including us, throughout the ages. Science calls it the CMBr or cosmic microwave background radiation. It is a field of electromagnetic or thermal radiation which vibrates at a range of frequencies. This field permeates our universe uniformly in all directions, at all times, and at all places at once with only relatively minor fluctuations. The CMBr connects all of creation.

The CMBr has recently been fully documented by the field of cosmology. Its frequency is modified in order to make it detectable by the human ear. However, the inner ear in the esoteric anatomy can detect the CMBr as it is found naturally in nature. The inner ear is not the physical ear canal. It is located at the occiput on the back of the neck.

The sound may initially be likened to the buzzing of bees, or the whistling wind. When listened to more closely, the sound is actually a bit complex. However, our mind tends to focus more on certain frequencies amongst the sound waves. This results in the select sounds an individual hears, such as the buzzing of bees or the whooshing wind.

Tinnitus is heard in the outer ear and results from damage to some of the cilia in the ear canal. The inner ear sound that we are currently discussing is heard at the back of the head, in the occipital area, where the skull and the cervical vertebrae connect. This is the inner esoteric ear. It is the placement of Da'at, the invisible sephirah in the body. Remember that the nature of Da'at is to connect to the entire universe. When an individual tunes in to the cosmic sound, they are stepping out onto a bridge which can connect them with all of creation.

At this stage a soul traveler may experience fear as they embark upon their journey. It is important to be able to release that fear. Always ask for protection and guidance from Ein Sof, our guide, or our higher power, prior to any meditation or soul traveling technique.

Even if we are not practicing the art of soul traveling, we can become still for a moment and listen. In that quiet we may hear a sound that was previously there but not consciously heard, like a gentle ringing or whooshing.

The sound that is heard in the inner ear can help connect us to the CMBr or cosmic microwave background radiation. Proof of the CMBr was sought after by cosmologists and, once documented, helped support the Big Bang theory. This frequency band stretches across our entire known universe and has done so for approximately 14.6 billion years or approximately 400,000 years following the Big Bang.

Ironically, unlike its name, the Big Bang itself was silent. The expansion of our universe contained only uniform radiation or light. There were no parts that were catching up with other parts, just pure light. There were no pressure waves and thus, no sound. Just a brilliantly silent, blinding glow of light.

As things cooled a bit and matter began to form from the light, matter dispersed in a way that contained slightly different densities that were due to quantum fluctuations. These minor fluctuations resulted in gravitational waves and oscillations that begat frequency waves. We now refer to this sound as the CMBr.

The ever so slight variations of the original wave patterns were insignificant in the early universe. However, with expansion, inflation, the impact of the CMBr, and gravity upon atomic matter, those slight variances were greatly amplified. The CMBr then continued to play its role in molding the structure of our universe as we know it today by way of its waves pushing on matter. These movements resulted in the structure of our known universe, including all of its stars, galaxies, planets and eventually, us.

It is that very cosmic sound that continues to envelop us individually and impregnates our entire known universe at the same time. It is this cosmic sound or set of frequencies that we seek to connect with or 'travel on' in our inner ear when we soul travel. When we are catapulted into what looks like space, it is through our actively connecting with a frequency that is uniformly distributed throughout space and time that we become one with the whole of the manifest universe.

We are ultimately one with all creation. Having the perception of being separate in our physical bodies is a personal experience that allows us to have the opportunity to grow and mature. In having a flash of our true nature, of our ultimate connection with everything while we are in the physical body, we are given the unique opportunity to expand our consciousness such that greater learning and understanding may take hold. This both benefits us as individuals and anyone we touch or work with as therapists.

Discovering the CMBr helps to prove an important aspect of what KST has been teaching all these years; that we're all one and that experience is both physically accessible and definable.

Remember that the physical World of Asiyah is a reflective vessel. That is why a unification experience is not an end within itself; It is a bridge by which we connect with the manifest universe. It is an imperative step toward accessing further levels of knowledge and experience.

Kabbalah states that we are only aware of one to ten percent of existence. Science reflects this by stating that all but three to five percent of the universe is known to us. Even the field of psychology says we are only conscious of three to five percent of our brain function and the medical field only claims to know that much about the physiological workings of the human body. The point is there is still so much of existence that is beyond our reach. That feeling of euphoric connection with the entire universe is only the beginning. Stay grounded and allow life's adventure to unfold.

By connecting with the cosmic sound, we raise our awareness to a more universal level. The breath becomes one with the body as the soul becomes conscious as one with the olamot worlds and beyond. This experience of universal connection enables us to be fully present in the moment, in our life and in our practice. The technique of connecting with the cosmic sound can be an effective and meaningful tool for therapists and bodyworkers for the purposes of healing and self-discovery.

It is imperative to remain grounded while this expansion of consciousness is occurring. Always remember that staying grounded during any meditative technique or experience is imperative to give that experience substance. Honor the mundane as much as the sublime, for ultimately, they are both the same.

Joseph Campbell said that the spiritual traveler and the schizophrenic swim in the same waters. The only difference is that the spiritual traveler can swim but the schizophrenic cannot. It's really a definition of level of functioning. As long as we can continue to function within the mundane day to day physical world, we can be free to explore the spiritual worlds without a problem. It is only when the spiritual becomes to us more important than the physical that we can get lost. Stay grounded and the universe can open to us. Lose that grounding and we may lose our way.

A side benefit to remaining grounded as a therapist and bodyworker is that we can be fully connected to our physical practice while simultaneously living in the sublime. This also helps to not take on the energy of our client. We provide a safe, therapeutic space to work and solid framework for healing to occur.

Merkabah

The merkabah is a three-dimensional representation of ZA. In two dimensions it is represented as the six-pointed star. It is a vehicle for soul traveling. The merkabah is mentioned at the end of chapter fifteen titled, "Color" and will be covered in detail in the next book.

CMBr AND KSMT MEDITATION

If the doors of perception were cleansed everything would appear to man as it is, infinite. [45]

—William Blake

Combining KSMT with the CMBr and merkabah enhances the soul traveling experience.

When we are able to soul travel, we facilitate expanded consciousness and, ultimately, experience a unification experience with our universe.

1. Sit comfortably and clear your mind. Contemplate oneness.
2. Play the CMBr soundtrack or listen for the CMBr in your inner ear.
3. Imagine sitting in the middle of a merkabah with the symbol Yud between your brows.
4. Perform RT for 5 to 10 minutes.
5. Maintain this meditative state for 10 to 20 minutes.
6. Clear your mind of the visualization and meditate for 5 more minutes.
7. Bring your consciousness back to the here and now.
8. Begin to slowly move your body. What was your experience?

KSMT along with the CMBr contributes to expanded awareness and aids counselors, therapists and bodyworkers in becoming fully present and energetically protected during their sessions.

The awareness of a universal connection is an amazing sensation, even if experienced for only an instant; that single instant of awareness is a part of the eternal now. By connecting with the eternal now we fully realize that we are all one.

In Closing

There are a variety of ways to connect to universal consciousness. KSMT is but one miraculous tool that aids us in potentially understanding and experiencing what already is our natural state of unity.

By consciously connecting with the cosmic sound via soul travel and meditation, we may become more aware of our connection with the entire universe and, thus, our true nature.

Part IV

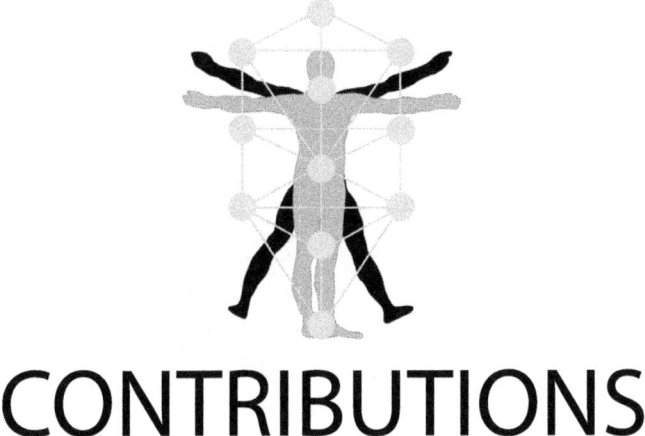

CONTRIBUTIONS

Chapter 17

KST Contributions

KST IS AN ORGANIC, EVER EVOLVING HEALING PARADIGM. A variety of fields help to define it. The papers below were written by a group of professionals who describe aspects of KST from the perspective of their designated field of study. It is with gratitude and awe that the following contributions are presented.

Sol Freidman, MA
Physicist / Musician / Artist

Sol is a brilliant, talented and multifaceted being. He has a master's in physics and a passion for music and audio. He does software consulting, art and enjoys writing and recording music. His work with the CMBr (cosmic microwave background radiation) relates directly to the Body of Atzilut in chapter eleven and the letter yud in chapter twelve.

The CMBr is the physical frequency that blankets our entire universe. It is a vibrating web of life. Techniques for the use of the CMBr in KST are described in detail in chapter sixteen.

Please enjoy Sol's written contribution to KST below:
"The CMBr or Cosmic Microwave Background Radiation is a snapshot of the early universe. It is the earliest picture we have

of the infant universe when it was around 400,000 years old. We cannot see any further back to the beginning of time, The Big Bang, because all matter was so hot that it was opaque to light.

This giant expansion of matter and light, and even space itself, created pressure waves that had a sound. We can recreate this sound by converting the CMBr picture so that we can hear what the universe sounded like at the very moment this "CMBr snapshot" was taken.

This conversion happens in a few steps. The variations in brightness of the CMBr tell us how loud each of the portions of the universe was. The size of the objects gives us the corresponding wavelengths, which we can convert into frequencies, or pitches.

The result: We hear the universe as it truly sounded as it was rapidly expanding into the universe we see today!

As a musician, working with the CMBr sound for KST was fascinating. It's sound is so organic and alive that when I attempted to change or process the sound, it took away the liveliness—it would accept nothing but its own pure original sound.

Nature speaks to us in strange and wonderful ways; it is said she speaks in the language of mathematics. This couldn't be more true here: the math and science that went into taking this picture of the infant universe and the math that it took for us to translate it into sound allows us to both see and hear this precious moment—the beginning of life for the universe and for us."

Gordon Goldberg, MA
Aerospace Engineer

Gordon Goldberg has been an integral part of many space and defense programs. Included are the Apollo missions, Israeli systems design, B1 Bomber and the Space Shuttle. During his service in the Korean War he received the Flying Cross. His profound accomplishments are balanced by his unfettered humility.

Below is Gordon's contribution to KST. It is a description of how light and matter translate to being the same substance in various states of frequency.

The mechanics of KST work with the physical body as frequency. The reference to orange light in chapter three is directly related to Gordon's mathematical breakdown of the orange fruit that follows.

Please enjoy Gordon's written contribution to KST below:
"To get a handle on the amount of energy held in a bit of mass, it's convenient to compare the energy produced by a one-hundred-watt light bulb. It emits ten times more heat than light, with a familiar object, say a three-ounce orange.

By $E=mc^2$, the energy contained in the orange would be about (0.8 x 1016) watt seconds, enough to power (0.8 x 1014) bulbs for one-second. If there are 200 million houses in the United States and each one has twenty-five bulbs inside, the orange could light them all for about 4.44 hours.

A few orange trees could provide for all our indoor house lighting every year, all year, with some left over to eat.
- $E=mc^2$ (Energy=mass x speed of light in kilometers per second squared)
- mass in kilograms
- energy in joules, 1 joule = 1 watt second
- Energy in a three-ounce orange is:
- $E=(3)(.03)(3x10)$"

John-Reid Theriac, MA
Geologist

John-Reid works in the oil and energy industries. His work has inspired a fascination with the interdependent workings of nature.

John-Reid helps make complex science accessible to the layman. Here is how he explains the use of crystals in KST as found in the next KST book, scheduled for release in 2021:

Please enjoy John-Reid's written contribution to KST below:
"Geology may seem mundane at times but it is the infrastructure that supports our life. We need to understand our relationship to this infrastructure in order to work with it in a realistic and sustainable way.

Crystals are an integral part of our environment. They are lattice like in structure that belies their mineral composition in a lattice-like form. Yet, their growth patterns follow that of many organic compounds. They could be said to exist between the inorganic and organic definition of life.

Crystals refract light and energy through their lattice like structures in a way that helps KST practitioners use them as a healing tool. The refraction of frequency is the same as x-rays that travel through the crystal latices. The frequency is then reflected or refracted by the physical characteristics of the crystal. The x-rays are a frequency traveling on a wavelength, like light. This is why you can take white light and distort it through a prism and create all the other frequencies (colors) of light in the rainbow.

Certain microscopes are bi-polar microscopes. This means they shoot the light through a type of filter. This means different minerals in the rocks will produce an increasing scale of color change. The amount of color change depends on how bi-polarable they are. The more bi-polar the mineral is, the brighter the colors will be. The more faded/pastel they are the less bi-polar the mineral is.

Another example would be sonar. Sonar is the measurement of how sound wavelengths are refracted or reflected off of objects. This measurement results in 3D image of the object.

All of these examples have to do with frequency. KST describes an energy body as a frequency, so it must travel in wavelengths. Those wavelengths will travel through the crystal lattice being used as a KST healing tool. They are refracted or reflected in some way that is aligning the ohrim with the sephirot. Then you can come to the conclusions that some crystals may help in creating a colorful prism of color on the wall or eradicate a dysfunction that could lead to disease."

Anne Weisman, PhD, MA, KSM, LMT
Director of Integrative Medicine, UNLV

Anne is exceptional in her field of holistic care. As the director of Integrative Medicine at the University of Las Vegas Medical School, she helps expose future generations to alternative medicines. She is a KSM practitioner, developed a protocol for performing a KST ToL reading from a distance, contributed two case studies and wrote the forward of this book. Her care, tenacity, brilliance and unbounded joy are grounded in experience.

She is a natural healer and was one of the first people to become a KSM practitioner. Anne continues to inspire and help all those she comes into contact with.

Gina de-Roma, KSM
Yoga Therapist

Gina DeRoma is a yoga therapist, bodyworker and KSM practitioner. She nurtures her numerous clients and helps heal all those she comes into contact with.

One of Gina's passions is conscious cooking. Her books and blog, "Philosophers Spoon," offer weekly healthy recipes with a dash of philosophy. Gina was the content editor for this book and previous KST manuals.

CHAPTER 18

Case Studies

THERE ARE TWO GENERAL TYPES of approaches to research. They are quantitative and qualitative research. Both have different purposes. Quantitative research is based on statistics. Qualitative research is primarily exploratory. The KSTechnique® case studies that follow fall under the descriptive qualitative research design category of research. They are meant to express the researchers observation of their own and their client's experience with KSTechnique® treatments.

WHY DOES KST EMPHASIZE CASE STUDIES?

OUR KSTECHNIQUE® COMMUNITY has remained small for the years it has been practiced. This was both by the intentional design of the founder and a natural result of lack of marketing. Jordania wanted there to be a small solid base of practitioners before it became more open. She knew that KST inspired her as her life's work. Then, it was up to the work to speak for itself and grow naturally.

Over the years there have been numerous positive outcomes reported from KSTechnique® treatments. Writing down some of these experiences into a case study format allows for congruent communication among practitioners. Writing down our experiences as case studies allows us to remember, build on experience and build a body of work to help establish the effects of this work.

What follows are a few examples of descriptive qualitative case studies based on naturalistic observation. They represent a variety of observational methods, experience and outcome and utilize a variety of writing styles and techniques. These differences reflect the diverse backgrounds and experience of KSTechnique® practitioners. Guidelines were not restrictive beyond case studies needing to be done as an in-depth investigation of the treatment course using KSTechnique® techniques.

It is hoped that these mini studies will lead to further research in the field of healing and integrative wellness. As we continue this work, our healing community will continue and expand its awareness of this work in an effort to gain a better overview of its impact and potential.

The case studies that follow deal with a full spectrum of client issues. The names and identifying descriptors of clients and patients have been changed. They include simple spa treatments, psychotherapy intake study, stage four cancer patient, and pets. These are but a few examples of many. This work is indicative of a great variety of circumstances in a multitude of venues. From them we can glimpse and experience the flexibility and efficiency inherent in KSTechnique.

Case Study by Dr. Anne Weisman, PhD, MA, KSM, LMT On Hospice, Death and Surviving Cancer

First hospice experience with KST

From the initial KST training, my practice has transformed. I work as a massage therapist for hospice patients. Throughout a typical day, I am working with people facing a variety of terminal diseases. In addition to each of the different patient's diagnoses, each individual has their own life experiences that they bring along. At the end of life, many issues surface. Massage therapy is beneficial and helpful for these patients. However, the addition of KST into the massage has been transformative. The first time I did KST with a patient was incredible.

I prepared myself to begin my rotation and thought about trying this modality with him. I felt strongly that this would help. I saw his family in the unit and asked if I could work with him to do the massage and KST I was learning. They informed me that he was no longer responsive but that I could work with him.

I knocked on his door and introduced myself again as I entered the room. After I washed my hands and prepared for his session, I thought through the sephirot and began to work with him. As I moved through the sephirot and came up to Binah, Chochmah, and Keter, his energy was noticeably different. At Keter, he began to laugh gently and I almost hit the floor.

I let him know I was with him and doing massage and energy work and at that moment, his dad flew around the corner as he heard his son's voice. We gathered bedside as he spoke briefly and told us he was "just having the best dream." I told him to return to it if he wished. He smiled and slowly drifted off. His dad and I remained with him for the next few minutes. I finished the session and the enormity of what just happened began to settle in.

I completed my day in the unit and as I was preparing to leave to go see my patients in home care, his nurse came into my office to let me know that he had just died with a smile on his face. I went to speak with his family and say goodbye. As soon as I was outside, I called Jordania to ask her what in the world did she teach me?!!?

I told her exactly what happened and she listened in her beautiful way. From that day on, this technique has been an integral part of my practice. I use it with my clients, teach it to my students and meditate with it to discover what is happening in my own body. Through the years of doing this technique, many other incredible things have occurred.

Another person I encountered early in my learning of this technique was a friend of mine who had recently been diagnosed with cancer. I was still learning the words and my Hebrew was rough. He patiently let me work with him as I placed flashcards on his sephirot and stumbled over the names and meanings. He has two children who would watch and listen to this each day that I would come over and do this work. They became my helpers and would place the crystals on their dad while we worked together. His journey through this particular bout of cancer led him out of state and it was then that we discovered that we could do this technique remotely.

I set my table as though he was coming in for a treatment and we picked the time to begin. I went through the whole session just as if he was laying on my table and the pendulum was picking up his energy! I took notes and recorded each reading. When the session ended, I called him and told him what the readings were. He and I were astounded as the readings were spot on. There was one particularly strange reading, of which I had never seen the pendulum move like this. We found out later that this was exactly where his cancer was. We did this work continually until he came back home and began to heal here.

KST brings the interconnectedness of our being back into focus. This technique can heal our world, one person at a time.

—Dr. Anne Weisman, PhD, MA, KSM, LMT, is currently the Director of Integrative Health at the Las Vegas Medical School in Las Vegas, Nevada. She is a KSM level practitioner. While working as a massage therapist, her work traversed spa and celebrity clients to hospice and stage four cancer patients. As the director the integrative medicine department at a medical school, she is helping transform our western model of medicine into a more integrative approach. Her work with our worlds future doctors gives hope that a holistic view of the body can become a natural part of our study of medicine as a whole. Anne continues to work and inspire others with her work as the director of integrative medicine at the University of Las Vegas Medical School.

Case Study by Aaron Nishimura, LMT, KSP
Soulful Journey

There was a strange vibe when I first picked up my client from the spa's waiting area. She tried to tell me all her issues at once jumping from one to another without completing an explanation. I could tell her emotions were all over the place. There was a tremble in her voice and it sounded like she would bawl at any moment. She did mention getting energy work in the past from Jordania, the creator of KSTechnique, our spa's Soulful Journey treatment. That was intimidating because Jordania's skill level and the time she spent practicing energy work far exceeded mine. Somehow, I hoped to meet my client's expectations. She wanted me to "do what I do" for the treatment and make her feel better. There was no specific request to work on a particular area or sephirot.

To show my intent to help, I decided to smudge the room with sage to cleanse the working area before beginning the treatment. While I sequenced through the four gates hold, she mentioned feeling much better. That put me at ease and gave me confidence that we could accomplish more in the 80 minutes. After completing the initial assessment, Sephirah 2, Yesod, had little pendulum movement. I did not mention this while going through the assessment and had the intention of letting my client know after completing all ten sephirah. Before I had the chance to comment on my observation regarding Yesod, she brought up Malchut and why that sephirot needed attention because of its association with being grounded. Analytically, that made sense based on our conversation and interaction so far. She immediately followed with another self-assessment that her "left side, the feminine side, is off."

The ten corresponding crystals were placed on or near each sephirot beginning with Malchut and ending at Keter. I have always used all ten crystals in prior Soulful Journey treatments and could not remember if I was originally taught to use only the corresponding crystals of the sephirah or sephirot focused on following the crystal placements. I applied the Earth Elemental Blend aromatherapy over Malchut and immediately followed with the corresponding earth energy (body points) hold. As with the crystals, all four elemental blends were used along with the related elemental holds. We were engaged in conversation throughout the crystal placement, elemental blend/energy holds, and the entire full body massage. The conversation seemed to distract my client, at least temporarily, from dwelling on the issues that were bothering her when she first entered the room. The 80 minutes flew by. Her crystal of choice to take home corresponded with sephirah 9, Chochmah.

There were a few steps I forgot to do and try. I forgot to play the CMBr. Blame it on the conversation. I also forgot to try the symbols Yud, Hey, Vav, Hey. Thank G-d I didn't need them this time. Also, I really did not elaborate to my client the assessment of any specific sephirot or the treatment as a whole at the conclusion. This is not my norm. We just got carried away with conversation this entire time. I was glad we connected and she did mention enjoying the treatment. I guess sometimes, people just need to be touched with positive intentions and have someone be an ear for whatever is on their mind.

—Aaron Nishimura has an extensive background in finance, massage and the healing arts. He is a licensed bodyworker and KST practitioner at Qua Spa in Caesars Palace, Las Vegas.

Case Study by Danielle Gilbert, LMT, KSG
Life Transitions

Client: 30-year-old male. Had been traveling around New Zealand, Australia and Indonesia for the last year. Moving to Boston for a *real job* in real estate and to put down roots for the first time in his adult life. Feeling excited about the new venture, though bittersweet to leave behind traveling adventures. Stopped in Las Vegas before heading to his new life.

Sephirot reading:
Malchut: erratic energy, counter-clockwise, right to left and left to right diagonal
Hod & Netzach: both right to left horizontal
Tipheret and Keter: wide open clockwise
Binal & Chochmah: counter-clockwise

I did reflexology to ground him as much as possible before working attachment points on knees and hips to open up channels of energy flow. Gentle stretching of the neck and energy encouraging cranial sacral work.

By the time I flipped him over, I reassessed the sephirot and all nine were wide open and clockwise. Air, Fire and Water oils were all used to help promote a balance of energy.

Client feedback, including note written on napkin:
After discussing overwhelming feelings of contentment and peace, we discussed strength in feeling grounded no matter where you are. He chose to leave with a hematite stone which represents the first, grounding Sephirot of Malchut.

"Danielle, I wanted to thank you again for my session today. I really believe that it was really beneficial to my state of mind at this particular time in my life. I think the treatments and service you provide for others is healing and invaluable. Thank you. I wish you the best in the future."
—Jonathan

It was interesting to see the energy change just by stating words and allowing him to process while assessing his energy. From the moment we met, I asked what he was looking for out of this treatment and why he chose it. Since he was making such a big move and committing to this huge shift, I knew Malchut would possibly be a little off. It was satisfying to know that some attention to Malchut could help put his mind at ease for this new chapter.

—Danielle Gilbert is a Midwife working through Balanced Birth Midwifery, Monitrice, Doula Services & Placenta Encapsulation. She is also a Licensed Massage Therapist of over eleven years. Danielle is a KSG level practitioner who continues to perform numerous KSTechnique® treatments at her full time spa position. As of the printing of this book, Danielle has begun an RN program.

Case Study by Eli Moran, LMT, KSG
Colors and Relaxation

This was a Soulful Journey treatment I performed at Qua Spa on April 16th, 2019.

I focused on Binah, the sephirah of understanding. I worked with the fire element and the symbol Hey.

The client's body alignment was off balance. The left shoulder was slightly elevated. The position of her neck muscles were shorter on that left side. Her right knee was very different from her left.

My client's body was vibrating at some point. Then, deep relaxation occurred in the middle of our session. The color of green was mostly present for me and the sound of a few tiny little bells that sounded as though the wind was moving through them from time to time.

I shared my experience of the session with my client. She did not see it or feel it exactly the same way. Her experience was different but really good.

My client felt amazing, relaxed and rejuvenated following our session. She said that she felt warm and so comfortable, like she was in her mother's arms and she was cradling her. In the very beginning my client spotted the color purple and then a star.

Sometimes I feel like I have to work extra hard on a client. But this was not the case in this session. The trust my client had in me to begin with was already a bonus.

I felt like I was able to aid in some conscious expansion for my client. I helped bring more awareness for grounding. This was necessary for her Binah.

The one challenge I came across was creating enough silence so that my client could hear the healing sound current we use during this treatment.

—Eli Moran won three Olympic medals, performed in Circ du Soleil, is a bodyworker and healer and has taught numerous seminars. She currently works as a licensed bodyworker and KST practitioner at Qua Spa in Caesars Palace, Las Vegas.

Case Study by Rabbi Jordania Goldberg: MA, KSM
Psychology of personal meaning

Referral Source: Rebecca was referred by her friend (my client), Sarah Jones. Names have been changed.

Client Referral Source statement of need and treatment expectations:

Sarah is concerned about Rebecca's recent depression and isolation following the loss of her 26-year marriage. Her expectations for treatment are that Rebecca would feel better about herself, find meaning in her life and get along better with her children. She would "like her friend back." Rebecca has not been exposed to holistic forms of psychotherapy and bodywork but the progress Rebecca has seen Sarah experience has let Rebecca to inquire about it during the last few months.

Presenting problems and situation:

Rebecca is a 53-year old woman who lives with her two teenage children. She is in the process of a divorce. Rebecca's husband moved out of their home three months ago. Rebecca has been married for twenty-six years to her high school sweetheart. They married shortly after she completed her bachelors' in chemistry. Afterwards, Rebecca began to work to support her husband through medical school. Upon her husbands' graduation Rebecca gave birth to their first child and became a full time stay at home mom. She reports she felt fulfilled with home life and her participation in the community. Approximately five months ago she caught her husband in a compromising relationship. He has since moved out of their home and has filed for divorce. Rebecca indicated she was deeply sad and upset about her husband's infidelity and "abandonment" of the family. Rebecca reports that she feels "lost."

Current Symptoms/Behaviors: (supported by DSM V diagnostic criteria):

Rebecca described her mood prior to her husband's infidelity as generally content and indicated it had gotten substantially worse since he left. Her affect was systemic during the assessment and she teared up several times. When I asked her what her intention was for her treatment, she asked to know what her purpose is as she feels untethered. She is also easily triggered, especially with her children and husband. Rebecca is experiencing sleep disturbance. During the week, when her children are occupied at school, Rebecca will sleep up to 11-12 hours. Self-esteem is poor. It was difficult for Rebecca to think of anything she likes about herself. She blames herself for not being "enough" for her husband. She has trouble connecting with her sense of self and purpose since, up until now, her identity was attached to her role as a wife and mother. Rebecca reported that she does not have much energy. She used to enjoy helping with her children's school and after school activities and coordinating her husband's schedule and social events related to his work.

For the last six months Rebecca has had excessive fears and worries. She denied panic attacks. She denied hallucinations, delusions, obsessions or compulsions. Rebecca denied problems with physical aggression. Activity level, attention and concentration were observed to be within normal limits. Rebecca denied symptoms of eating disorder. Rebecca reported some recent weight loss.

KST Assessment:

Rebecca's affect was curious but reserved about the holistic portion of the assessment. Rebecca's primary constitution is earth and water. The water influence is accentuated from her sign of Cancer and is exacerbating the earth imbalance in the form of depressed mood of a diatomic quality.

Tree of Life reading was as follows: Keter (open), Chochmah (open), Binah (cut off), Chesed-Yesod (blocked), Malchut (confusion). Rebecca's connection with what she wants in her life to look like is clear. When she attempts to intellectualize that ideal it is blocked—cut off from her emotions and core sense of self. This cut off may be leading to confusion in her sense of stability. Rebecca agreed with the reading. She wanted further guidance as to what steps to take to feel better and get to know how she was as an individual apart from her marriage and role as a mother.

Psychiatric Treatment History:
Rebecca reported that when she was about ten-years-old she saw a counselor during her parent's divorce. She reported that she found the past counseling helpful, however, she only saw the counselor a few times and is not sure why her mother stopped taking her. In retrospect she wonders if it was part of a psychological assessment for some of the court proceedings her parents were undergoing at the time.

Substance Abuse Treatment history:
None reported.

Recent (30 days) alcohol and drug use:
Rebecca reported that she has been drinking a "couple" of glasses of wine per day during this month. She indicated that it helps her to relax and cope. Onset of this behavior began shortly after her husband announced he was leaving and was going to file for divorce.

Current Medication Regimen:
None reported.

Medication allergies/adverse reactions:
Rebecca reported she has seasonal allergies. There are no known allergies or adverse reactions to psychotropic medications.

Family and Social Status: (current & historical):
Rebecca's husband left the family six months ago. Rebecca continues to live in her home of twenty years with her two children, a thirteen-year-old boy and a sixteen-year-old girl. Rebecca's social circle mostly consists of other mothers in her area who have continued to reach out to her and are sympathetic to her plight.

Rebecca's mother lives forty-five minutes away and has stepped in to take care of things at home and with the children when needed. Rebecca has two younger sisters, both of whom live too far away to help with her directly, however, they are available on the phone for emotional support. Rebecca's father passed away from a heart attack ten years after he left the family, when Rebecca was twenty years old. Rebecca had just gotten engaged to her husband when her father died. Rebecca reported that her husband (then fiancé) could not handle Rebecca's feelings of grief and abandonment and he almost broke off the engagement. Rebecca chose to deny her feelings of grief in order to placate her husband-to-be. This pattern of denying her feelings in consideration of her husband's expectations continued throughout their marriage.

Rebecca reported a 'normal' childhood. There were no problems with her as an infant that she is aware of and she was told that she achieved developmental milestones on time.

Rebecca is sometimes uncertain about how to manage her feelings about her divorce. Although she is adept at denying her feelings she is choosing to try and face them since they have become overwhelming. Rebecca reports concern about the welfare of her children. Her son is "shut down" and her daughter shows signs of sadness and anger and sometimes verbally accosts Rebecca, telling her that 'it is her (Rebecca's) fault that their father left.' This only further mirrors Rebecca's belief that her husband left them because she was "not enough." Rebecca's daughter's outbursts shock her since Rebecca choose to be silent when her parents got divorced.

Since their separation, Rebecca has only communicated with her husband regarding child and financial issues. Rebecca reports that when her husband first announced that he was leaving she began to cry and plead with him. Her husband's response became detached and cold. His response triggered Rebecca to stop her feelings in the hopes that it would make things okay. Her husband left anyway and Rebecca was left in a state of "shock" and a feeling of being "lost."

Rebecca reports crying but only while she is alone. She has attempted to act as though everything is okay for the sake of her children, however, she is finding it more difficult to "manage" her daughter's outbursts. Rebecca reports that she doesn't understand why her daughter can't "hold it together" the way her brother is and the way that Rebecca did when her own parents got divorced.

Legal Status:
Currently Rebecca is separated for six months. Rebecca received divorce papers from her husband last week. Her husband is not seeking custody of their children. Rebecca has had no legal violations.

Vocational/Educational Status/Functioning:
Rebecca completed her bachelor's degree in chemistry prior to getting married. Once she was married, she worked as a pharmaceutical representative in order to help put her husband through medical school. Once she was pregnant, she stopped working and became a full-time homemaker and mother. When asked about childhood aspirations she said that up until her parents' divorce at the age of ten she wanted to be a ballerina. Afterwards, she lost touch with her dream.

Current Community Resources and Services:
Rebecca is actively involved in the community Temple. She is active in her children's school. These activities appear to continue to be a support for Rebecca and her children. Rebecca has wondered whether to see a psychiatrist of psychotherapist. When she asked her friend Sarah what was helping her, Sarah told Rebecca that she had been coming to see me for a series of six treatment sessions and it had been beneficial. Sarah suggested that this form of holistic psychotherapy might also benefit her. Rebecca has also consulted with other friends during this time.

Personal and Social Resources and Strengths:
Rebecca has some insight into her problems and is motivated to change. She is feeling lost. She is not certain what her purpose is beyond wife and mother and would like the opportunity to explore that. She has a good community network and a few close personal friends, who are

also mothers. For the last six months Rebecca has found it difficult to interact with her support network and attend to her commitments. Her current living situation appears to be stable and financial resources appear adequate. Her husband has stated that he will continue to financially support her and their children.

Diagnostic Impression:
DSM: 309.21 (F93.0) Separation Anxiety Disorder, Single Episode, Mild to Moderate Dependency.
KST: Keter (open), Chochmah (open), Bina (cut off), ZA(blocked), Malchut (confusion)
Sign: Cancer
Element: water and earth
Applicable psychotherapy techniques: Rogerian Argument and congruency, Satires roles for family systems

Treatment Plan:
Based on Rebecca meeting the criteria for DSMV's Separation Anxiety Disorder, I would recommend she commit to an integrative approach that incorporated both psychotherapy techniques and KST treatment.

Based on the psychotherapeutic basis of KST assessment I would utilize the Rogerian Argument to help integrate her ideal self to her core self. The KST assessment shows that this is possible by opening the channel within Binah to allow the current flow of Keter to integrate into her sense of self. The KST assessment showed that the Supernal Triad and Malchut, although there was confusion in Malchut, were all open, only blocked at Binah as it connects to Zer Anpin. This shows a dissociation between Rebecca's mental processes and her emotions. Helping Rebecca become aware of herself, her emotions and teaching coping skills to express those emotions and communicate them congruently will lead to a productive outcome with her children and community. Energy work would include the earth protocol to help ground these processes.

Based on the element of water and Rebecca's water and earth constitution, I would recommend a lifestyle balanced for water and earth respectively.

The treatment plan was discussed with the client. All questions the client had were answered to her satisfaction.

Rebecca asked to complete a series of treatments to better practice and integrate this treatment plan.

GLOSSARY

THIS GLOSSARY DEFINES WORDS that appear in the text and some common words associated with Kabbalah that have specialized meaning when used in KSTechnique. No attempt is made to give the range of meanings beyond those used in the text. For fuller definitions and other shades of meaning please consult a standard dictionary of Kabbalah or psychology.

KSTechnique® Terms

Abraham - Patriarch associated with the Sephirah of Chesed.
Aaron - Patriarch associated with the Sephirah of Hod.
Aether - One of the five elements. It is associated with the tip of the Hebrew letter Yud and the reflex zones in the body.
Air - One of the five elements. It is associated with the Hebrew letter Aleph, Air Constitution, shoulders, sides, ankles and torso in the body.
Alignment - Proper body structure. To be in harmony with the letters.
Angel - Messenger. Temporary force of nature.
Archangel - Permanent and named angel.
Archetype - A model of first form that becomes a universal symbol of the human unconsciousness. Jungian principal.

Attenuation - Slowing of frequency and quality of the ohrim as it progresses through creation. The reduction of the amplitude of a signal, electric current, or other oscillation.

Archetypes - Universal representations of psychological processes. Carl Jung developed the concept of archetypes in conjunction with the collective unconscious. Both archetypes and the collective unconscious are pertinent to the level and Body of Atzilut. Carl Jung's archetypes were based on Plato's Forms.

Asiyah - Lowest level of creation. Relates to Body of Asiyah (physical body) (or Zelum Elochim) and the Final Hey.

Attunement - To come into alignment with the letters as symbols.

Atzilut - Fourth level of creation. Relates to Body of Atzilut (spiritual body) and Yud.

Avir - Energy field that extends from an individual or structure.

Beriah - Third level of creation. Relates to Body of Beriah (mental body) and Hey.

Big Bang - Scientific theory of the evolution of the universe.

Binah - Understanding.

Binah Consciousness - Level of functioning that resembles traits of Binah.

Bittul - Self-transcendence.

Body Alignment - Consciously aligning the body for the best structural efficacy.

Body of Atzilut - Spiritual body. Relates to the level of Atzilut and the letter Yud.

Body of Asiyah - Physical body (or Zelum Elochim). Relates to the level of Asiyah and the Final Hey.

Body of Beriah - Mental body. Relates to the level of Beriah and the letter Hey.

Body of Yetzirah - Emotional body. Relates to the level of Yetzirah and the letter Vav.

Bodies of Avir - Energy bodies that are extensions of an individual or structure that has a ToL as its core structure.

Chesed - Love.

Chesed Consciousness - Level of functioning that resembles traits of Chesed.

Chochmah - Wisdom.

Chochmah Consciousness - Level of functioning that resembles traits of the Sephirah of Chochmah.

CMBr - Cosmic microwave background radiation. A field of electromagnetic radiation or frequency that permeates our known universe.

Collective Unconscious - The term was coined by Carl Jung. In KST is also describes our unconscious on the level or Body of Atzilut.

Collective Consciousness - Jungian principle of psychology where human consciousness is connected within a collective. It's language is that of archetypes.

Cohesive Consciousness - State of being that contains spiritual virtues.

Collective Unconscious - Psychological principal made popular by Carl Jung. Refers to the collection of shared material within the human psyche which take the form of archetypes within the unconscious.

Da'at - Knowledge. Invisible sephirah.

Dermis - Middle layer of skin.

Distillation - Process of essential oil extraction using a solvent.

Earth - One of the five elements. It is associated with the Hebrew letter Hey, Earth Constitution, neck, colon knees and feet in the body.

Ego Consciousness - Ego as "I" is central to functioning.

Ein Sof - Infinite. Without end.

Energy Construct - A section of anatomy, physiology or psychology of the esoteric anatomy. To set in logical order particular parts of the esoteric anatomy or physiology.

Enfeurage - Essential oil extraction without using heat. Plant material is washed in alcohol or placed on a fatty surface.

Epidermis - Top layer of skin.

Expression - Peel of (usually) citrus is scratched or smashed between rollers in order to extract the essential oil from the pith. Then a certifying machine separates the pure essential oil.

Esoteric Anatomy – Anatomy of the energy field.

Esoteric Psychology – Psychology of the energy field.

Esoteric Physiology – Physiology of the energy field.

Final Hey – Power symbol.

Fire – One of the five elements. It is associated with the Hebrew letter Shin, Fire Constitution, forehead, solar plexus, thighs and head in the body.

Formless Point – Tip of Yud.

FP – Formless point.

Gabriel – Archangel associated with strength. Associated with the left side of the body.

Gematria – Numerological system by which Hebrew letters correspond to numbers.

Gevurah – Restraint / severity / judgment.

Gevurah Consciousness – Level of functioning that resembles traits of Gevurah.

Heart-Mind – Secondary placement of Binah is the heart. Binah's knowledge becomes the intelligence and fire of the heart.

Hebrew Letters – Part of an ancient and modern language whose letters can be used as symbols in KSTechnique.

Healing Crises – The body experiences an illness or imbalance on its road to health. This usually occurs when stuck energy in the body begins to move out of the body.

Hertz – Measure of frequency in number of oscillations per second.

Hey – Mental symbol.

Hip Circles – Facilitates movement of Yesod energy in the body.

Hip Shimmy – Facilitates movement of Netzach and Hod energy in the body.

Hod – Splendor.

Hod Consciousness – Level of functioning that resembles traits of Hod.

Hydrodiffusion – Similar to steam distillation, except that the steam enters at the top of the still.

Hypodermis – Deepest layer of skin.

Inhalation of Essential Oil - Process of absorbing an essential oil through the breathing airways. Also, breathing.

Issac - Patriarch associated with the Sephirot of Gevurah.

Jacob - Patriarch associated with the Sephirot of Tipheret.

Joseph - Patriarch associated with the Sephirot of Yesod.

Kavana - Intention.

Keter - Crown.

Keter Consciousness - Level of functioning that resembles traits of Keter. Consciousness associated with feeling full, bright and expansive.

King David - Patriarch associated with the Sephirot of Malchut.

KSH - Kabbalah Somatic Hold.

KSMT - Kabbalah Somatic Meditation Technique. A meditative technique that aids the practitioner or client in achieving a more unified, peaceful or transcendent state of consciousness with the aid of the CMBr sound.

Maceration - Plant material is quickly placed unto hot fat or other absorbent material which is then washed with alcohol that evaporates leaving the volatile essential oil.

Latent - Unknown or inaccessible.

Makif - Surrounding light.

Malchut - Kingdom.

Malchut Consciousness - Level of functioning that resembles traits of Malchut consciousness of emptiness that reflects judgment based on the physical universe.

Maya (downward) - A figure eight movement made by rolling the hips outward one at a time. This facilitates movement of sephirotic energy from Keter to Machut in the body.

Manifest - Becoming known or accessible.

Mate-ve-lo-mate - Truths that exist in contradiction of each other.

Maya (upward) - Facilitates movement of Sephirot energy from Malchut to Keter in the body.

Merkabah - Six-pointed star in three dimensions. A vehicle of soul travel.

Michael - Archangel associated with compassion and love. Works with the right side of the body at the level of the Sephirah of Chesed.

Middot - Emotions. The six sephirot of Zeir Anpin are called middot.

Moses - Patriarch associated with the Sephirah of Netzach.

NDR - Near death experience.

Netzach - Victory.

Netzach Consciousness - Level of functioning that resembles traits of Netzach.

Olam Murgash - World of emotions.

Olam Muskal - World of thought.

Olamot - One of the four (or five) layers of existence called worlds or universe.

Ohr Ein Sof - Infinite light.

Ohrim - Healing light of Ein Sof / universal life force.

Ohr Ein Sof - Infinite light.

Panimi - Internal light.

Partzuf - Anthropomorphic representation.

Raphael - Archangel associated with healing and back issues. Works with the spine and nerves.

RT - Breath technique based on the concept of ruah hakodesh.

Ruah Hakodesh - Breath of life.

Sechel - Hebrew word for Intellect. The supernal triad are called Sechel.

Sephirot - Energy center. The building blocks of the worlds and universe.

Shoulder Shimmy - Connects Chesed and Gevurah energy to the body.

Snake Arms - Facilitates movement of Chesed and Gevurah energy in the body.

Tetragramaton - Combination of four Hebrew letters used for healing in KSTechnique. These letters as symbols are associated with the five worlds.

Tipheret - Beauty.

Tipheret Consciousness - Level of functioning that resembles traits of Tipheret.
Torso Circles - Facilitates movement of Tipheret energy in the body.
Walking Camel (downward) - Facilitates movement of sephirotic energy from the Sephirah of Keter to the Sephirah of Malchut in the body.
Uriel - Archangel associated with enlightenment and moving forward in life. This energy works with the front of the body.
Universal Consciousness - Conscious connection with the universe.
Vav - Emotional symbol. Hebrew letter with a gametria of six.
Vessel - Forms within creation that are able to contain spiritual light.
Vessel Consciousness - Our ability to contain spiritual light.
Walking Camel (upward) - Facilitates movement of sephirotic energy from the Sephirah of Malchut to the Sephirah of Keter in the body.
Soul Traveling - Movement of the soul into a more universal experience.
Steam Distillation - Essential oil extraction using steam.
Teshuva - Taking correct action toward healing.
Tikkun - Rectification of the light. Fulfilling our life's purpose.
Transcellular - Through the cells.
Transdermal - Through the skin.
Tzimtzum - Kabbalistic theory of the evolution of the universe.
Water - One of the five elements. Water is associated with the Hebrew letter Mem (Water Constitution), the chest, pelvis and feet in the body.
Yesod - Foundation.
Yesod Consciousness - Level of functioning that resembles traits of Yesod.
Yetzirah - Level of creation above Asiyah or the physical world. Relates to Body of Yetzirah (emotional body) and the letter or symbol of Vav.
Yud - Healer of the soul.
Zelum Elochim - Energy body that is the blueprint for the Body of Asiyah (physical body).

BIBLIOGRAPHY

Chapter 1
1. Ralph Waldo Emerson: Quotes.
2. Albert Einstein: Quotes, 1954.

Chapter 2
3. Son Nakagawa: Quotes.
4. Albert Einstein: Quotes.

Chapter 3
5. Matt, Daniel C. *Zohar: Pritzker Edition, Volume IV*, California: Stanford University Press, September 28, 2007.
6. Kaplan, Ayreh. *Sefer Yetzirah: The Book of Creation, Revised Edition*, 1:5, p. 44. 665 Third Street, Suite 400, San Francisco, CA 94107: Weiser Books, San Francisco, CA / Newburyport, MA. Revised edition published in 1997 by Red Wheel/Weiser, LLC, www.redwheelweiser.com. 1997, Copyright @ 1997 The Estate of Aryeh Kaplan.
7. Kaplan, Ayreh. *Sefer Yetzirah: The Book of Creation, Revised Edition*, 3:4, p. 51. 665 Third Street, Suite 400, San Francisco, CA 94107: Weiser Books, San Francisco, CA / Newburyport, MA.

Revised edition published in 1997 by Red Wheel/Weiser, LLC, www.redwheelweiser.com. 1997, Copyright @ 1997 The Estate of Aryeh Kaplan.

8. Kaplan, Ayreh. *Sefer Yetzirah: The Book of Creation, Revised Edition*, 1:6, p. 51. 665 Third Street, Suite 400, San Francisco, CA 94107: Weiser Books, San Francisco, CA / Newburyport, MA. Revised edition published in 1997 by Red Wheel/Weiser, LLC, www.redwheelweiser.com. 1997, Copyright @ 1997 The Estate of Aryeh Kaplan.

Chapter 4

9. Kaplan, Ayreh. *Sefer Yetzirah: The Book of Creation, Revised Edition*, 3:4, p. 57. 665 Third Street, Suite 400, San Francisco, CA 94107: Weiser Books, San Francisco, CA / Newburyport, MA. Revised edition published in 1997 by Red Wheel/Weiser, LLC, www.redwheelweiser.com. 1997, Copyright @ 1997 The Estate of Aryeh Kaplan.
10. Rabbi Scherman, Nosson, Rabbi Zlotowitz, Meir. *Psalms* (104:5), The ArtScroll Series / Stone Edition / The Tanach, p. 1527. 4401 Second Avenue / Brooklyn, NY 11232: Mesorah Publications, Ltd., August 1999.
11. Chidvilasananda, Gurumayi. *Paraphrase from meditation intensive:* Oakland, California, Siddah Ashram, 1983.
12. Matt, Daniel C. *Zohar: Volume IV, Pritzker Edition*, p. 402, Stanford, California: Stanford University Press, September 28, 2007.
13. Anodea Judith, p. 83.

Chapter 5

14. Matt, Daniel C. *Zohar: Pritzker Edition, Volume IV*, p. 382, #54. Stanford, California: Stanford University Press, September 28, 2007

15. Rabbi Scherman, Nosson, Rabbi Zlotowitz, Meir. *Psalms* (104:1), p. 1527, The ArtScroll Series / Stone Edition / The Tanach. 4401 Second Avenue / Brooklyn, NY 11232: Mesorah Publications, Ltd., August 1999.
16. Matt, Daniel C. *Zohar: Pritzker Edition, Volume V*, p. 158 (2:123b). Stanford, California: Stanford University Press, 2009.

Chapter 6

17. Matt, Daniel C. *Zohar: Pritzker Edition, Volume IV*, p. 382. Stanford, California: Stanford University Press, September 28, 2007.

Chapter 7

18. Matt, Daniel C. *Zohar: Pritzker Edition, Volume IV*, p. 382, Stanford, California: Stanford University Press, Stanford, September 28, 2007.
19. Matt, Daniel C. *Zohar:* Pritzker Edition, Volume IV, Pritzker Edition, p. 130 #223. Stanford, California: Stanford University Press, September 28, 2007.
20. Matt, Daniel C. *Zohar: Pritzker Edition, Volume IV*, p. 372 #11. Stanford, California: Stanford University Press, September 28, 2007.
21. Kaplan, Ayreh. *Sefer Yetzirah: The Book of Creation*, Revised Edition, 3:4, p. 38. 665 Third Street, Suite 400, San Francisco, CA 94107: Weiser Books, San Francisco, CA / Newburyport, MA. Revised edition published in 1997 by Red Wheel/Weiser, LLC, www.redwheelweiser.com. 1997, Copyright @ 1997 The Estate of Aryeh Kaplan.
22. Thoreau, Henry David; Introduction/Merwin, W.S. *Walden and Civil Disobedience,* first chapter/Economy: Signet. The Mass Market Paperback edition, 2012.
23. Kaplan, Ayreh. *Sefer Yetzirah: The Book of Creation, Revised Edition*, 3:4, p. 40. 665 Third Street, Suite 400, San Francisco,

CA 94107: Weiser Books, San Francisco, CA / Newburyport, MA. Revised edition published in 1997 by Red Wheel/Weiser, LLC, www.redwheelweiser.com. 1997, Copyright @ 1997 The Estate of Aryeh Kaplan.

Chapter 8

24. Kaplan, Ayreh. *Sefer Yetzirah: The Book of Creation, Revised Edition*, 1:4, p. 38. 665 Third Street, Suite 400, San Francisco, CA 94107: Weiser Books, San Francisco, CA / Newburyport, MA. Revised edition published in 1997 by Red Wheel/Weiser, LLC, www.redwheelweiser.com. 1997, Copyright @ 1997 The Estate of Aryeh Kaplan.
25. Campbell, Joseph. *Myths to Live By: Chapter X, Schizophrenia - the Inward Journey*. 375 Hudson Street, New York, New York 10014, U.S.A.: Penguin Group, Penguin Putnam Inc., Copyright @ Joseph Campbell, 1972.

Chapter 9

26. Kaplan, Ayreh. *Sefer Yetzirah: The Book of Creation, Revised Edition*, 1:7, p. 57. 665 Third Street, Suite 400, San Francisco, CA 94107: Weiser Books, San Francisco, CA / Newburyport, MA. Revised edition published in 1997 by Red Wheel/Weiser, LLC, www.redwheelweiser.com. 1997, Copyright @ 1997 The Estate of Aryeh Kaplan.

Chapter 11

27. Matt, Daniel C. *Zohar: Pritzker Edition, Volume IV*, p. 360, #37. Standford, California: Stanford University Press, September 28, 2007.
27. *Isaiah* (43:7), p. 1527, The ArtScroll Series / Stone Edition / The Tanach, Edited by Rabbi Nosson Scherman, Published by Mesorah Publications, Ltd., August 1999.
28. Matt, Daniel C. *Zohar: Pritzker Edition, Volume IV*, p. 408, #143.

Stanford, California: Stanford University Press, September 18, 2007.
29. Kaplan, Ayreh. *Sefer Yetzirah: The Book of Creation, Revised Edition*, 1:2, p. 22. 665 Third Street, Suite 400, San Francisco, CA 94107: Weiser Books, San Francisco, CA / Newburyport, MA. Revised edition published in 1997 by Red Wheel/Weiser, LLC, www.redwheelweiser.com. 1997, Copyright @ 1997 The Estate of Aryeh Kaplan.

Chapter 12

30. Matt, Daniel C. *Zohar: Pritzker Edition, Volume IV*, p. 431, #228. Stanford, California: Stanford University Press, September 28, 2007.
31. Matt, Daniel C. *Zohar: Pritzker Edition, Volume I, Tosefta*. p. 381. Stanford, California: Published by Stanford University Press, October 28, 2003.
32. Matt Daniel C. *Zohar: Pritzker Edition, Volume V*, p. 160 (2:123b). Stanford, California: Published by Stanford University Press, 2009.

Chapter 13

33. Kaplan, Ayreh. *Sefer Yetzirah: The Book of Creation, Revised Edition*, 3:6, p. 150. 665 Third Street, Suite 400, San Francisco, CA 94107: Weiser Books, San Francisco, CA / Newburyport, MA. Revised edition published in 1997 by Red Wheel/Weiser, LLC, www.redwheelweiser.com. 1997, Copyright @ 1997 The Estate of Aryeh Kaplan.
34. Matt, Daniel C. *Zohar: Pritzker Edition, Volume IV*, p. 407, #140. Stanford, California: Stanford University Press, 2009.

Chapter 14

35. Rabbi Scherman, Nosson, Rabbi Zlotowitz, Meir. *Psalms* (104:1), p. 1527, The ArtScroll Series / Stone Edition / The Tanach. 4401

Second Avenue / Brooklyn, N.Y. 11232: Mesorah Publications, Ltd., August 1999.
36. Matt, Daniel C. *Zohar: Pritzker Edition, Volume V*, (2:98b) p. 29, #81. Stanford, California: Stanford University Press, 2009.
37. Matt, Daniel C. *Zohar, Pritzker Edition, Volume V, (2:98b)* p. 29, #82. Stanford, California: Stanford University Press, September 28, 2007.

Chapter 15

38. Matt, Daniel C. *Zohar: Pritzker Edition, Volume III*, p. 404. Stanford, California: Stanford University Press, December 5, 2005.
39. Color / Define Color at www.dictionary.com.
40. Rabbi Scherman, Nosson, Rabbi Zlotowitz, Meir. *Genesis* (1:3), p. 3. The ArtScroll Series / Stone Edition / The Tanach. 4401 Second Avenue / Brooklyn, N.Y. 11232: Mesorah Publications, Ltd., August 1999.
41. Matt, Daniel C. *Zohar: Pritzker Edition, Volume III*, p. 471. Stanford, California: Stanford University Press, Stanford, California, December 5, 2005.
42. Kaplan, Ayreh. *Sefer Yetzirah: The Book of Creation, Revised Edition*, 1:7, p. 57. 665 Third Street, Suite 400, San Francisco, CA 94107: Weiser Books, San Francisco, CA / Newburyport, MA. Revised edition published in 1997 by Red Wheel/Weiser, LLC, www.redwheelweiser.com. 1997, Copyright @ 1997 The Estate of Aryeh Kaplan.
43. Matt, Daniel C. *Zohar: Pritzker Edition, Volume III*, p. 473. Stanford, California: Stanford University Press, December 5, 2005.

Chapter 16

44. Albert Einstein: Quotes, 1954.
45. William Blake: Quotes.

Additional References

Einstein, Albert: "Ether and the Theory of Relativity" (1920), republished in *Sidelights on Relativity* (Methuen, London, 1922)
http://cds.cern.ch/record/358722
https://www.nature.com/articles/168906a0
http://cds.cern.ch/record/515241/files/0108217.pdf
https://arxiv.org/abs/1203.6655

Additional Sources

Wise, Michael & Abegg Jr., Martin & Cook, Edward. *The Dead Sea Scrolls, A New Translation*, Broadway, Published by HarperCollins Publishers, 2005. Chapter 36, The Book of Enoch, New York, NY, p. 280.

Savedow, Steve. *Sepher Rezial Hemelach: The Book of the Angel Rezial.* York Beach, Maine: Samuel Weiser, Inc., 2000. P. 7.

Wikipedia. Sefer Raziel HaMalakh. Internet: wikipedia.org.

Brett & Foer, Joshua. *Separia:* Lockspeiser, Internet: sefaria.org., (Maimonides) Mishneh Torah (circa 1180), 2011. *A Dictionary of Angels by Gustav Davidson, Encyclopedia of Angels by Richard Webster, The Complete Encyclopedia of Angels by Susan Gregg, The Encyclopedia of Angels, Second Edition by Rosemary Ellen Guilty, The Encyclopedia of Angels by Victoria Briggs.*

Brett & Foer, Joshua. *Separia:* Lockspeiser, Internet, Talmud (Tractate Rosh Hashanah 1:2), 2011.

ABOUT THE AUTHOR

RABBI JORDANIA GOLDBERG, MA, KSM is the founder of KSTechnique® (KST).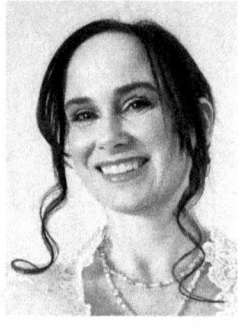

This groundbreaking, healing modality is a culmination of Jordania's life's work. Her background in teaching, counseling, psychology, bodywork, Kabbalah, Ayurveda, Reiki, Polarity, Cranial Sacral Therapy, meditation, art, healing and dance are all heart-felt passions that helped create a structure for the inspiration of KST. Jordania maintains a virtual counseling practice and continues teaching KST seminars while working on the second part of this book. She is also the creator of two small holistic product lines—Sankaya and OM7.

www.ingramcontent.com/pod-product-compliance
Lightning Source LLC
Chambersburg PA
CBHW071219080526
44587CB00013BA/1424